ELEVATING MASCULINITY -

The POWER of MEDITATION for MEN

...♦...

Transform Your Mind,
Transform Your Life

Noraa Casi
and
Ray Nebado

TABLE OF CONTENTS

—◆—

INTRODUCTION

—◆—

If you're reading this book, then you have made a smart decision. Perhaps you have experimented with meditation before, and now you need some guidance, or maybe you're thinking about taking it up for the first time, but you need more information. Whichever it is, I can guarantee that you're about to learn everything you need to know—and not just about how to meditate.

Now, it's very probable that the readers of this book will be in different life stages; not necessarily dependent on age, but rather circumstances. And the good news is that you can all derive great benefits from meditation. Indeed, you will definitely get to know yourself better, and in doing so, you will operate more effectively in a way that promotes mental wellness.

Meditation is more complex than you might think; in fact, it takes years of practice to master the art. However, at the beginning, even if you are only able to meditate for 30 seconds before becoming distracted by thoughts, don't worry. That is completely normal, and also completely okay. If you manage 30 seconds, that's better than nothing at all, and in any event, you don't need to stop there. You can refocus by clearing your mind of all thoughts and getting back to the task at hand.

You may have heard of mindfulness before, and that's good because it's going to be a big theme in this book. Mindfulness goes hand in hand with meditation and is all about being present in the moment. The former can be differentiated from the latter in terms of presence. Again, like meditation, it may take you some time to get going. However, mindfulness is easier to get better at than meditation, even though both practices have the same—or, at least similar—outcomes. There are many ways in which mindfulness can be used, and as you continue reading, you will gain the knowledge to use it on a daily basis—and not only when you sit down by yourself. We tend to go through life without paying any mind to the monotonous things, like waking up in the morning and getting ready for work. This is where mindfulness comes in. It teaches you to observe your surroundings in greater detail, aided by your senses, to draw enjoyment—and distraction—from the simplest sights, sounds, tastes, and general activities you experience. And when I say "distraction," I'm talking about a good kind. When you're distracted in a good way, there is little time to dwell on negativity, stress, anxiety, and other feelings that impair your well-being.

So, the first thing we have to do is make sense of what it means to be a "man" in society, as, at this point, you may be struggling to reconcile manliness with meditation. I hope you agree—and if not right now, I'm confident you will in good time—that there are stereotypical ideas of manliness, which society expects us men to adhere to. However, you should be comfortable enough in yourself to tell friends and family that your meditation practice doesn't make you any less of a man. To that end, we are going to address the myths surrounding meditation, and we will also look at the stories of highly successful men who have benefited greatly from meditation. Success, whatever that may be for you, can be the result of inspiration from people who have achieved incredible things, and as such, it can be the first building block to your success.

All people have a feminine and masculine "operating system." Men have an internal masculinity, and so do women, although the latter has smaller doses. The opposite is also the case, and as you and I both know, males and females differ in their approaches to life. For instance, masculinity is often associated with strength, stoicism, problem-solving, and a need for competition. Now, many of these traits are true of men, but not always. As we continue, I will explain more about male and female social interactions, which will assist in learning about yourself. For the moment, though, I am going to pose a question, and I want you to answer it, and see if it changes your mind. There is no wrong answer, and at this stage, it's really just an opinion: *Should we challenge toxic masculinity?*

All humans are complicated, and an interesting theme on this score is shame and its origins—as well as its relevance. If you have ever felt shame, and are confused about the reasons behind your shame, I'm going to help you gain a better understanding. As men, we tend to suppress our emotions more than women, and on the point of shame, not dealing with related emotions can be particularly damaging to our mental health. Forgiveness falls into this category, and holding onto grudges has no benefit to either party. On that note, you will learn about how meditation and mindfulness can help you forgive others *and* yourself. Are you starting to see how vast the concept of meditation is?

Meditation can be helpful for stress, emotional resilience, cognitive improvement, memory, and clear thinking. When you synergize all of these benefits, you can get the most out of both meditation and mindfulness. Breathing is a big component of each, and in Chapter 7, we will go over a series of important breathing exercises to aid in these areas. Whether you've heard of them or not, we're going to go over alternate nostril breathing, the 4-7-8 method, and pursed lip breathing, along with box breathing, mindful breathing, and lion's breath. Breathing fills your blood with oxygen and releases carbon dioxide, so the general gist of deep breathing is to maximize oxygen intake and maximize carbon dioxide release... you'll see what I mean. I referred to "synergy" earlier, and what that essentially means is that all parts of something operate together. Your aim, then, is to create synergy between the different components of your mind and body, and when everything is working together, you will know—and it will be wonderful.

The subject of journaling may be one you are uncomfortable with, but it's something that's going to require attention. Sitting down with a pen and some paper, with no distractions and an allocated time, has the potential to lead you to a greater understanding of yourself, as a person, and as a man, which is why we will discuss self-discovery through mindfulness and meditation. Remember that positive affirmations, identifying problems, and discovering areas of your life that you would like to improve upon are instrumental in the development of mental sharpness, clarity, and good decision-making. To identify your true self, you need to consider a wider consciousness, work on emotional intelligence, and engage in self-reflection.

Have you ever heard the acronym, "S.M.A.R.T."? Well, it refers to a framework you can apply to your goal-setting, which is used often in the business and corporate world. Specifically, it's concerned with shedding any ambiguity from your goals. For instance, "I want to be rich," is such a broad, vague goal, that it's almost bound to be unattainable. In particular, using the word "want" is not part of S.M.A.R.T. because, well, it makes you *want* something instead of *work* for it. Don't worry, S.M.A.R.T. is a simple concept that you'll pick up easily, with obvious benefits for not only setting but *reaching* your goals. Trust me, getting uncomfortable can make you more comfortable; I will explain that concept in good time.

Mindfulness stretches as far as communication. With that in mind, I'd like to pose a challenge to you: Before you get to Chapter 6, wherein we'll be discussing communication more thoroughly, try to work out what mindful communication may look like. Do some roleplay with a friend or family member in regard to the way you think mindful communication should be held. This isn't a test, but by the time you reach the end of that chapter, you'll know if you were correct or not.

The body-mind connection is not one that necessarily involves a physical aspect. On that note, progressive muscle regulation is not an exercise—rather, it's a manifestation of muscle use as a means of stress relief. The body is also involved in the mindfulness scan, and again, though it's not an exercise, it does build a synergy between mind and body—just from a focus standpoint as opposed to a physical exertion one. Have no fear—these concepts will become clearer when we discuss reliance and resilience-specific meditation techniques in further detail.

Lastly, we're going to finish off with some useful tips on how to practice meditation, consolidating all the overall benefits—including mindfulness. The tips are both simple and actionable and will grant you that last bit of motivation needed to get going, and to continue along your journey of personal growth.... and so, all that's left to say is: *Let's go!*

CHAPTER 1:

Understanding Men - What Does It Mean to Be a Man?

—◆—

I could probably write a whole book to answer the above question, as truly, it could be answered in so many ways. For one, you have the "Cowboys don't cry" opinion, which is almost certainly outdated. Perhaps a more contemporary view is that men can be strong and sensitive at the same time. And then, of course, a certain portion of the older generation may believe that being a man means being a provider, which may be true, but that doesn't mean a woman can't occupy that very same role.

If you had to ask Thomas Paine, the 18th-century Founding Father, politician, and philosopher, he would have said that, "I love the man that can smile in trouble, that can gather strength from distress, and grow brave by reflection. 'Tis the business of little minds to shrink, but he whose heart is firm, and whose conscience approves his conduct, will pursue his principles unto death" (Brainy Quote, n.d.).

Let's break that down. Smiling in times of trouble doesn't mean that you're *immune* to the trouble. But it does mean that you have the right attitude, which is to accept that there are problems and make an effort to find solutions while carrying yourself in a positive manner. Indeed, nobody has ever sailed through life without hardship, and the way you deal with your own hardships is what reflects on you as a human being. Gathering strength from distress may be interpreted as an act of stoicism, but it also goes to the heart of putting in the work needed to pull yourself out of the space of distress in your personal circumstances.

Reflection is a wonderful tool for motivation, as with it, we can use the past to inform our future decisions. Also, remember that your arguments will determine your reality. This is an especially important point, which we will explore further as we progress through this book. Maybe Thomas Paine's definition of what it means to be a man is not the same as your definition. However, upholding your values, being true to yourself, learning from your mistakes, and striving to be the best version of yourself—no matter your definition—are virtues that should form part of your approach to life. And now that we've given life and opinion to Paine's words, this is what you can expect from the remainder of this chapter:

- an overview of how manliness is perceived by society
- how the notion of masculinity has evolved
- stereotypes among men in wider society
- cultural stereotypes
- getting to know yourself better

With this agenda, I am to give you an accurate idea of traditional, progressive, and perhaps even narrow-minded conceptions of being a man.

What Does Being a Man Mean in Society Today?

It would be impossible to speak with every single adult on the planet to get an overall view of what manliness is. However, there are trends—especially in Western society—that can give us a relatively accurate idea. This is best done by breaking down masculinity into three categories. But before we do, I would like to give you the dictionary definition, as follows:

> *The fact of being a man; the qualities that are considered to be typical of men (Oxford Learners Dictionary, n.d.).*

Next, we're going to look at three categories of so-called "masculinity," ranging from those characterized by more toned-down qualities to those that can be considered over-the-top or even outright dangerous.

Soft Masculinity

This type of manliness is characterized by greater personal care, an interest in fashion, and the ability to tap into what would previously have been considered feminine. Now, soft masculinity doesn't mean being overly sensitive or turning away from manly pursuits. In fact, a man who is a bodybuilder, football player, or boxer, and—for lack of a better word—is considered "macho," can still take part in these self-care qualities. Indeed, moisturizing, conditioning, and tapping into spirituality will not make you less of a man. Let's look at another example: Some men are of the opinion that it's their responsibility to open doors for women or stand up when a woman arrives at a meeting or coffee date. Furthermore, certain men may feel threatened if a woman objects to this type of treatment, citing it as outdated chivalry. These are, of course, just examples, but they are the best way to illustrate soft masculinity.

Positive Masculinity

Men in this category display the old-school traits of strength, bravery, and courage, in addition to paying attention to the sensitivities of others. As such, they're generally caring, motivated to help others, and, to be blunt, they're "prepared to change the diapers," no longer seeing this as the sole job of the mother.

Toxic Masculinity

One of the first words that come to mind when talking about toxic masculinity is *misogyny*. Indeed, men in this category believe women to be subservient, holding to the belief that women, in a sense, belong in the kitchen. They think of themselves as dominant figures, void of weakness, with an elevated sense of self-importance. I think it's fair to say you want you to steer clear of this type of masculinity. Lastly, Andrew Tate has become the figurehead for toxic masculinity, and if you haven't heard of him, give him a quick Google search, and you'll discover just how terrible toxic masculinity can be.

Before we move on, please keep in mind that the above three categories of traits are not mutually exclusive, and can exist in conjunction with each other.

Traditional Stereotypes

When it comes to masculine stereotypes, a lack of mental health concerns is quite common. The traditional idea is that *emotional* toughness must be accompanied by *mental* toughness, and furthermore, sensitivity must not be shown at all. It's not that men don't have emotions, though; it's just that they don't show them—nor even accept them. As a result, males essentially wear masks to hide their inner feelings. Another stereotype is that men should be in control of women, no matter the context. As with mental health awareness, though, this is also changing—perhaps not fast enough, but we'll get there. The reality is that as long as gender differences exist—and they always will—stereotypes will be around too. However, with societal progress—hopefully aided by books just like—some of those stereotypes may just change for the better.

Cultural Stereotypes

Now, masculinity, of course, looks different in different parts of the world. Some may say that the West is more advanced due to the ways in which equality is prioritized. Indeed, men are equal to women, and there are no two ways about it—except there are. As for certain non-Western cultures, though, they see masculinity, the roles of men, and the roles of women, through a completely different lens. In cases where women are oppressed, perhaps they know no better, or accept that their religion, culture, creed, or any other factors are just the way things are, and thus this subservience is normal. This can be a challenging topic, of course, because outsider opinions on manliness in these cultures may be considered unfounded; then again, it's a matter of opinion.

From there, we have to ask what the role of the man is in *religions*; say, Christianity, Judaism, Hinduism, Buddhism, and even other niche religions that follow spirituality. Perhaps these religions are not directly persecutory when it comes to women, but there has always been a traditional attitude that men are the strong, tough, stoic providers in families that follow these faiths.

Another group to consider is modern hunter-gatherers, and here I use the term "modern" to describe the times, and not necessarily the limited infrastructure that hunter-gatherer tribes have created. The Inuits, for example, remain hunter-gatherers, as do the Mbuti people in the Democratic Republic of Congo, and the Kets of Siberia.

Ultimately, we can sum up all these cultural stereotypes by saying that they lean toward the "men provide, women stay at home" archetype. For the hunter-gatherers, the stereotype is true, but the women in those communities have equally important jobs and are equally as tough. The same could be said of modern cultures wherein women are seen as suppressed. It is, however, safe to say that at the heart of every culture, there is a stereotype that men must be strong, emotionless, and in charge. Please remember, though, that stereotypes don't apply to everyone, and just because they exist as perceptions, this doesn't mean they have truth to them.

Self-Discovery, Acceptance, and Growth Through Understanding Masculinity

Human beings are complex creatures, and you, the reader, are no different. Some people go through their whole lives without truly coming to terms with who they *really* are. Masculinity, in its stereotypical form, may have something to do with that because introspection may not be seen as *manly*. However, if you can truly discover yourself, and accept what you discover, then you have taken the first steps to personal growth.

Therapy is one form of achieving growth, and contrary to what some may say, it actually takes strength to stand up, admit that you need help, and commit to whatever means will facilitate that help. When it comes to self-discovery and acceptance, there are many ways to embark on that journey. In a nutshell, you need to take a look at yourself—an honest one. Indeed, you need to identify the good bits *and* the bad bits, accept them without self-judgment, and work on rectifying those bad bits while maintaining control over the good ones. When you're able to be more honest with yourself, you lay bare parts of yourself that you've tried to suppress, and through that, you promote vulnerability. The good news is that from vulnerability comes growth, and as we continue, you'll learn a lot more about how meditation can help with self-discovery, acceptance, and growth.

Meditation, Masculinity, and Mindfulness

If we fall back on stereotypes, we may think that meditation has no space or limited air time for men. But the thing is, meditation is so much more than sitting cross-legged and slowly chanting some phrase. For one, as you know by now, it incorporates mindfulness. Again, meditation and mindfulness are not the same thing, but they do overlap in a significant way.

You should remember from the Introduction that mindfulness is defined by presence, while meditation is defined by calm. The reason for this differentiation is that mindfulness is based on the ability to stay focused on the present moment, while mindfulness can be practiced in a wider context. Indeed, mindfulness can be practiced through several mindfulness exercises that don't require you to close your eyes as you would while meditating. The basic principle is to be focused on the present, and through that focus, be absent of thought, worries, stress, and anxiety. Like the other concepts we have dealt with briefly in this chapter, meditation and mindfulness will each be addressed in more depth as we continue. For now, you just need to know that the two concepts *can* defy stoicism, and furthermore, they can challenge the idea that men should be emotionless.

Chapter Takeaway

With this first chapter done, I'll leave it to you to make up your own mind in regard to that Thomas Paine quote we analyzed earlier. When it comes to masculinity, though, know that there are three broad categories: soft masculinity, positive masculinity, and toxic masculinity. The latter is the one to avoid, but the other two have their merits, without a doubt. Strong and sensitive fit together, as do toughness and self-care, which together can break down the traditional ideas of what masculinity actually is.

Traditional stereotypes, of course, are largely based on the standing of men versus the standing of women in society, and although there has been a widespread historical notion that men put food on the table, it is women who have always prepared that food. And from there, more progressive attitudes are observable in the present.

Cultural stereotypes are curious because many of them don't attract negativity, while others do, but from those not well-versed in that culture or those who have a different point of view. In any event, and no matter what culture, *new* masculinity means getting to know yourself, and showing vulnerability in the pursuit of personal growth.

Lastly, as we discussed, meditation is one way to garner growth and is often accompanied by efforts to stay in the present, otherwise known as mindfulness.

Now, going back to stereotypes for a brief moment, it's time to break some of them wide open. Indeed, as we move on to the next chapter, we will be discussing the feminine side of masculinity.

CHAPTER 2:

Embracing the Feminine in Our Masculine

—◆—

The true strength of a man is not measured by how forcefully he conquers others, but by how gently he cares for those around him.
–Unknown

Before we delve into the *why* and *how* of meditation, let's talk about the reasons as to why the masculine quality—in both men and women—may lead men to thinking that meditation is not "for" them.

Now, we could break down the meaning of conquering others, as per the opening quote. Does it mean a physical fight? Being better at sports? Being more intelligent? Doing well in business compared to competitors? Ultimately, though, it could mean any of the above, but what is more important is the second part of the quote. Being caring is the domain of all humans, or, at least, it should be. And in this case, I think we could apply the exact same quote to women—and even children. First of all, having people to care for is a wonderful thing, and being able to care for them in a kind and loving way makes one a good human. With these thoughts in mind, here is what you can expect from this chapter:

- the complexity of gender
- observable traits of men and women, both similarities and differences

- emotional intelligence and empathy
- problem-solving, logic, and analytical thinking
- relationship dynamics, and the idea of community
- binary assumptions and the impact of hormones

The Evolution of Masculinity

Many people say that chivalry is dead and that polite men are hard to come by. I completely disagree, first of all. A better way to characterize this scenario is to say that there was a time when men were expected to provide for women. Indeed, if we go all the way back to the hunter-gatherer days, the women did the work in their dwellings, and the men went out to hunt. There is a practicality to that; just by nature, men are stronger and faster than women, so it has made evolutionary sense that this primitive arrangement worked in the way it did. If we fast-forward many centuries to, let's say, the 1950s, the focus was on the wife making the husband happy, and the husband making the money. That is no longer the case, of course, and there is a strong argument to be made that modern masculinity is now about *equality*. A man can support women's rights, and in the same breath, he can be comfortable with his wife or girlfriend earning more money than him, and furthermore, being able to financially support herself. The subject is open for discussion, though, and there are many other factors to consider. Not all societies are the same, after all, and masculinity has evolved differently, depending on where in the world you live... we will get to that.

Redefining Masculinity

The English language could probably do without the word "masculinity," but it would no doubt be replaced with something similar. I say this because I don't think we should be compelled to define a term with one sole meaning. And the same can be said for gender. Over the last decade, the concept of gender as a spectrum has become a much more acceptable thing to discuss. There are, however, dangers associated when it comes to the way that children and teenagers may be influenced through content creators and media figures glorifying the idea of gender fluidity. We are seeing more and more transgender teenagers having surgery before they are even old enough to drive a car. Teenagerhood is a confusing enough time as it is *without* the complications of surgery, and while I fully acknowledge that you might be in the wrong body, it's probably best to wait until you are a young adult before making a decision so big that it will affect you for the rest of your life.

Among these realities there are many questions that pop up, but that aside, all of us need to show kindness when interacting with people we see as different. A man can be feminine, a woman can be masculine, and vice versa. Looking after your skin, reading magazines traditionally targeted at women, and taking an interest in hobbies that would be seen as feminine are some prime examples. The latter could involve playing sports associated with men or having weightlifting gym routines, which one would traditionally consider a man's domain. In fact, a man can be both masculine and feminine, as can a woman. The spectrum is wide, and within the different classifications on the spectrum, there is also a wideness. When I say that human beings are complex, *I mean it*.

Now, before we move on, I would like to share the "competitor versus creator" concept, as a tenet of masculinity, or perhaps expected masculinity. What it means is that despite the masculine tendency to compete and win, there should also be a focus on personal growth and improvement. Of course, these two metrics are measured against oneself and can support a shift from the competitor to the creator type of mindset. This would mean that it doesn't matter what anyone else does—your focus should remain on creating your own reality. Indeed, this should be your ultimate goal.

Typical Traits of a Woman

Real progress will only really be made once society gets to a point where we can talk about typical traits of people without outright separating men from women. At this point, society *does* differentiate, which is also okay, but it should not be so rigid when it comes to stereotypes. Women are seen as more nurturing, and that may not be wrong, because, from an evolutionary point of view, women are the ones who give birth, thereby creating that immediate nurturing bond. That being said, men can also be nurturing. In this same vein, women are generally expected to be compassionate, but we would hope that *everyone*, irrespective of anything else other than being a *person*, would display compassion. I hope you agree with me when I say that at the heart of the matter, there is no such thing as typical traits of any specific group. Unfortunately, though, societal stereotypes often paint a different picture.

Emotional Intelligence and Empathy

Certain people are highly intelligent when it comes to IQ, while others are intelligent in a book-smart way, and others, still, have both or neither of those traits. You get individuals who are good problem-solvers, who are successful in business, or who lead a nomadic lifestyle, digitally, or otherwise. Any or all of these types of individuals may lack emotional intelligence, but what does that even mean? Basically, it refers to the way we deal with people, meaning how we show kindness, help our fellow humans, and consider their own individual struggles. A boss who shows empathy when you tell them you're struggling with an issue at home has good emotional intelligence, but a boss who says something like, "I'm sorry to hear that, now get back to work," is displaying no emotional intelligence whatsoever. If you're concerned that you might lack emotional intelligence and are unable to empathize, then meditation—and its ally, mindfulness—are likely not activities you've considered engaging in.

From a masculinity point of view, if you are of the opinion that emotional intelligence and empathy are traditionally female traits—but you possess them, as a man—then you are not losing your masculinity. Rather, you are embracing it by caring for those around you, as the chapter-opening quote revealed. Furthermore, along with emotional intelligence and empathy comes a notion of community. You can empathize with anyone, from the cleaner to the CEO, no matter what differentiates you. Honestly, when you strip everything else away, we are all *humans*. Working toward bettering ourselves and society together, as well as making an effort to understand each other, are marks of emotional intelligence that offer a well-rounded type of masculinity. On top of that, embracing sensitivities, dealing with emotional sensitivity, and being willing to discuss one's feelings are all part of being emotionally intelligent, and men should not fear these things, just as women should not fear them. In fact, being emotionally available and vulnerable in a romantic relationship can go a long way in the success of that relationship.

Typical Traits of a Man

Just like with women, we shouldn't really have this category for men, and furthermore, we could quite easily get rid of it. We could even combine it with the typical traits of a woman to make an all-encompassing category that focuses on humans as humans, without any gender divide or any other source of division. Assertiveness and leadership could be traits attributed to men, but there is no reason why women cannot have the same traits. In fact, in reality, *they do*. A well-rounded man embraces both strength and emotional awareness—and again, so does a woman. "Manly" men are associated with fast cars, symbolism such as lions or eagles, and an expectation of fearlessness without emotion. Yes, some men are like this, but no—not all men are—or should be—like this.

Analytical or Empathetic?

The idea that men are more prone to analytical thinking is actually true, and in the face of research, we can't label the facts as sexist. Cambridge University collected data from nearly 700,000 men and women across the spectrum of race, religion, socio-economic standing, and age. The results backed the theory that men are more analytical, as well as more likely to understand rules-based systems, whereas women are more empathetic and better at understanding the emotions of others.

With this in mind, it's useful to bring up and differentiate between sympathy and empathy. The former is when you're able to look at someone's adverse circumstances, feel sorry for them, and make that known. The latter, in contrast, involves you experiencing the same emotions that they do instead of simply feeling sorry for them. This occurs because you identify with what they are going through. For instance, a parent and child bond could be seen as an example of "automatic empathy." Indeed, seeing your child in emotional pain is a trigger for you, as a parent, to feel the same emotional pain. And on that note, it could be argued that women have more of a proclivity for empathy because of the biological reasons discernible in motherhood. A 2021 study into the empathy activation areas in the brain found exactly that: mothers indeed displaced more brain activity, and this suggested more empathy than can be found in women without children (Irene Sophia Plank et al., 2021). All of that aside, men and women can be analytical, empathetic, both, or neither. However, problem-solving skills can be learned, as well as the ability to put oneself in another's emotional shoes and genuinely feel what they are feeling.

Competition

When it comes to feeling challenged, far more men are likely to become competitive than women. Indeed, among men, there is often a need to come out on top, no matter how silly or insignificant the subject of the competition. This is because men inherently play to win. In a more serious context, the workplace can be a competitive environment, and studies suggest that men are more competitive than women when it comes to their jobs in particular. Does this mean having a competitive nature is part of being masculine? Maybe, but again, as with the other areas of masculinity we've looked at, not everyone abides by the stereotype. From a research angle, in 2019, Harvard Business Review published the results of a large-scale study into competitiveness in males versus females, and the manner in which the research was done is certainly worth examining (Kesebir, 2019):

Researchers began by asking 111 men and 119 women to identify which parts of the competition they considered to be positive, and likewise, which parts they felt were negative. After looking at the results, it was decided that in order to create both a positive and a negative category, three subcategories would have to emerge, as follows:

- Positive
  - performance booster
  - character development
  - innovative problem-solving
- Negative
  - potential unethical behavior
  - damages self-confidence
  - hurts relationships

Now, I believe these subcategories do a fine job of summing up the pros and cons of competition. And in particular, I would like to point out that unethical behavior is often seen in sports, as a means to win in highly competitive environments. The most classic example is perhaps that of Lance Armstrong, the former professional cyclist who used performance-enhancing drugs to become arguably the best cyclist the world has ever seen. That is a topic for another day, but is nonetheless a very good example of one of the negatives of competition.

After having established what I will loosely refer to as a "metric," researchers asked 1,189 men and 1,142 women, specifically about competition and performance. 63% of the women were less convinced than the average man that competition boosts performance, builds character, and leads to innovative solutions. The findings in terms of feelings toward the negative metric were relatively even, but all things considered, the obvious conclusion was that men see more of a positive side to competition than women do.

Hormones

We humans are hormonal creatures, and all day, every day, our brains and bodies are producing hormones, which keep us operational. Naturally, then, hormones dictate our characteristics, as well as how we act. However, they also control bodily functions, including the following:

- physical development and growth
- metabolism
- sexual function, reproductive growth, and health
- cognitive function
- body temperature maintenance

With the above hormone-controlled functions in mind, let's have a look at the different ways in which hormones affect men and women.

Estrogen and progesterone are the major female sex hormones, which men also produce, but in much smaller quantities. Meanwhile, testosterone is the major male sex hormone, but again, women *also* produce it—just in smaller quantities. Hormonal changes and deficiencies can have negative sexual side effects, but the impact on our cognitive function, for the purposes of this book, is most important when it comes to how beneficial meditation can be.

Ultimately, both men and women experience hormonal shifts that can impact mental health. Stress, especially in the form of major life events like losing one's job, grieving the loss of a loved one, or any other sudden and unexpected change, can create hormone shifts that affect cognition. This can then result in anxiety, depression, OCD, and bipolar disorder. These four mental health conditions are sometimes dealt with by taking prescription medication and/or attending therapy sessions. Now, to bring us back to meditation and mindfulness, these two habits have proven instrumental in improving mental well-being. As such, they are optimal practices to bring into your life to aid in clinical conditions—as well as just in general.

So, we know that hormones are not the only thing that shape our personalities. However, men who have higher testosterone levels are more prone to aggression, more competitive, and have escalated sex drives, which one could say is the definition of toxic masculinity. Then again, I am generalizing, but for the sake of completeness, I would like to look at nonhormonal influences on personality, whether you are male or female (Ferguson, 2022):

- Genes
  - We have our parents to thank for our genes, and that is why we often share personality traits with

them.

- Life experiences
    - Abuse or neglect as a child, to use two obvious examples, could cause isolation and withdrawal as parts of your personality.
- Adverse events
    - Losing a loved one at an early age, being forced to flee your home due to a natural disaster, or having a major negative financial setback are major occurrences that have the potential to shape—and also change—your personality.

Without a doubt, it comes down to the "nature versus nurture" conversation. And when it comes to hormonal influences and life circumstances, there is always a balance, just not always an *even* one.

Feminism for Men

You don't have to be gay to advocate for gay rights, and you don't have to be transgender to advocate for trans rights. Following that thought pattern, you don't have to be female to be a feminist. The world of toxic masculinity might disagree, but that world still subscribes to women being subservient.

Although women and men are just about equal in our modern age, especially in most Western societies, announcing that you are a feminist as a man could get you some funny looks (which it really shouldn't). One side of feminism is self-care, although, of course, equal rights have been at the center of the feminist movement for decades. When we looked at soft masculinity in the previous chapter, I gave you the example of a football player who moisturized. Now, it could be seen as narrow-minded to say that self-care is part of feminism, but the point is that manliness can definitely involve self-care, and furthermore, is not a sign of weakness nor a sign that you are too in touch with your feminine side. A man who respects women—and sees himself as equal to any woman—is more of a man than one who sees women as subservient. On the other hand, being threatened by women, feeling the need to have a better job and make more money than women,, and wanting to be the sole decision-maker of the household, all make up an outdated view of masculinity. We can actually dispense with masculinity or femininity altogether as labels, and just be comfortable with who and what we are. Again, this is easier said than done, but practice eventually makes perfect.

Promoting Equality

Again, equality is absolutely a part of feminism, and as I've just said, a man who embraces gender equality is more of a man than one who practices misogyny. Then comes the argument of the traditional structure of the patriarchy, and how males should be involved in dismantling it. Debates have raged about what the patriarchy *actually* is, but in simple terms, it is the "man is the head of the household" school of thought. That is, of course, a very limited definition, but the patriarchy, in a broad sense, is responsible for the unequal distribution of power between men and women. Furthermore, the influence of the patriarchy can be seen in the government, in numerous businesses, and in many homes. Indeed, across the board, the patriarchy represents the exercise of power in several broad situations, with the common theme of men being the ones "in charge." The modern man— and I suspect you know what I'm going to say—is the type of individual who sees government, business, and home as places where equality between men and women should 100% be present.

Embracing Feminism

After everything you have read up until now, I hope that you will indeed embrace feminism, or at the very least, accept that men can be in touch with their feminine side, stand up for equal rights, and oppose the patriarchy. To do all of these things, you can't be *half in*. In fact, if you are going to embrace feminism, you have to be *all in*. And more than that, you should be proud of yourself for doing so.

Should We Challenge Toxic Masculinity?

The answer is, obviously, yes—and I'm sure you'd agree. However, this doesn't mean you can just go out into the street, looking for men who appear to embrace toxic masculinity and try to change their minds. There are other ways to counter this kind of toxicity.

One of the most appropriate examples involves the belief that if a man has many sexual partners, he is worthy of praise, but when a woman is in the same position, it's deemed morally objectionable. That, right there, is toxic masculinity in a nutshell. Indeed, it isn't the business of anyone else if you choose one sexual partner on a long-term basis, or prefer more sexual partners over the short term. It's also not the business of anyone else to be judgmental against either sex for these choices. Rights are arguably at the crux of the matter here, and toxic masculinity seeks to create more rights for men than women, which can also be said of the patriarchy, as discussed previously.

Ultimately, toxic masculinity—whether in relationships, friendships, or even in family circumstances—can negatively impact one's mental health. If a woman is made to feel controlled in a relationship, she is probably being affected by toxic masculinity. It's also highly possible that her partner makes her feel as though she's not good enough, or is in constant competition, and these things are absolutely signs of toxic masculinity. If you think that there's a crossover between toxic masculinity and toxic friendships, you are on the right track. Toxic friendships are often the result of one party once more asserting himself in a disproportionate way. If you suspect that you may uphold toxic masculinity but want to change, or you're a victim of toxic masculinity in a friendship, it's important to remember that with a bit of work, the situation has great potential to be altered for the better.

So, yes, we should challenge toxic masculinity.

Chapter Takeaway

Masculinity is definitely deserving of a new definition. While it may be true that women are more empathetic, and men are more analytically minded, this isn't a reflection on masculinity or femininity, which are traits that can coexist in both men and women. Men are more inclined to embrace competition, but that too doesn't define masculinity. There is a hormonal consideration, and hormones certainly influence the way you "are," but your environment also plays a role. Furthermore, as we've covered, a man can be a feminist and still be masculine. It would be fair to say that the balance of power, in several contexts, is shifting, and as much as we need to challenge toxic masculinity, we need to promote masculinity inequality too. On that note, it's time to get into meditation in greater detail, so, please join me as we discuss the *why* of meditation—among other subjects—in the next chapter.

CHAPTER 3:

Meditations for Men - Benefits and Examples

—◆—

Why should men be constrained by antiquated stereotypes of masculinity? What does it even mean to 'Be a Real Man' anymore? Shouldn't we all be celebrating a wide range of definitions of manhood?
–Andy Dunn

I'm sure that you'd agree with Andy Dunn, and answer his questions by saying that we should not be constrained, that you don't know what "real" is, and that a wide range of definitions should be celebrated. Why, then, do so many of us fit into, or try to fit into what we know is a stereotype, and in many cases, not one that is productive when it comes to our mental health? Well, in most situations, it's because we think that "this" is expected of us, or "that" is expected of us when, really, we should be true to ourselves and live our lives the way that we want to live them. So, if you find yourself subject to this kind of scenario, just remember that at the very least, you are exploring meditation, mindfulness, and related practices that work with one's state of mind. However, you may still see meditation as something that men "just don't" do. If so, then in this very chapter I'm going to change your mind. Indeed, we are going to take a look at several stereotypes and misconceptions, after which I guarantee you will be ready to embrace meditation and harness all the positivity that it can bring to your life.

Debunking Myths

If there are myths, there have to be realities as well, and if we can break apart those myths so that they're no longer seen as realities, then we are achieving something truly positive. To do so, though, you have to have an open mind and be prepared to live your reality without the adulteration of myths.

Meditation Is Only for Women

Now, we can cast the net wide, and say that in ancient times, sun or rain worship was a form of meditation. We can even say that the simple act of staring into a fire counts, and we most certainly still do that today. If we look at meditation as we know it, then we can point to various men who are accredited with its development in different regions. These men include the Hindu monk, Swami Vivekananda; the Buddhist monk, Hsuan Hua; the Christian friar, Saint Francis; and many others. As you can see, meditation is essentially pioneered by men—so truly, how could the practice not be seen as masculine? Well, this could be the product of society, and the machismo that has become associated with men. But while women have proven to be good at meditation, and have derived its benefits, so have men, and so you can absolutely become one of the latter. Many world-famous and influential men use meditation on a daily basis, and it is these public figures who can help us change this myth. Some examples are Kobe Bryant, Sting, Hugh Jackman, Jerry Seinfeld, and one of the greatest musicians ever, who had this to say about meditation:

It is a lifelong gift. It's something you can call on at any time. Now it's actually coming into the mainstream. I think it's a great thing.
—*Sir Paul McCartney*

Indeed, if Sir Paul McCartney is a passionate advocate of meditation, it's safe to say that we are heading in the right direction.

People Who Meditate Are Passive and Weak

Quite the opposite is true, actually. It's a bit like therapy: There is a long-standing opinion that seeking therapy makes you weak, and even more so if you're a man. On the contrary, though, admitting that you need help—and doing something about it—actually makes you *strong*. And we can say the same thing about meditation. It is, without doubt, a form of therapy, and modern psychology and psychiatry actually incorporate many elements of meditation in their practices. Individuals who seek out meditation may do so to quell their aggression, but at the end of the day, meditation is for your benefit and nobody else's, so if someone is telling you that you're passive and weak, but at the same, you're improving your physical and mental well-being, then they are clearly wrong. As human beings, we should be doing the things we can to look after ourselves, and there is *nothing* passive or weak about that. Ultimately, meditation is empowering, and all we have to do is look at the world-famous, profoundly successful men in the previous myth category to know that.

Meditating Conflicts With What It Means to Be a Man

Let me give you another example of something often deemed "unmanly" that is worth debunking: yoga. The practice has gained popularity over the last few decades, and while a large contingent of society tends to see it as a pursuit for women, it has actually been instrumental in also helping men with their physical health.

We have to remember that even before the stereotype situation occurs, there is also an *expectation* of the stereotype. So, though the similarity between yoga and meditation is the focus on breathing, that is beside the point. What I am getting at is that the thought, "a real man doesn't do yoga," finds its way into the minds of men in the same way that the thought, "a real man doesn't meditate," does. Ultimately, each thought has missed what being a man is actually all about.

This takes us back to Andy Dunn's quote, and his words ring especially true here. At the risk of repeating myself—but with the necessity to do so—we should be questioning *who* or *what* a real man is. Eating steak, drinking beer, swearing, talking down to women, and always trying to be "the man" are no longer appropriate parts of the definition. At the end of the day, meditation can help you become a *better* man, and to call on the opening quote, we know that a real man smiles in trouble, gathers strength from distress, and grows brave from reflection. All three of these virtues can be promoted through meditation, and no male is less of a man because he meditates. Don't forget that.

Men Must Not Express Emotion

I would say that this is only half a myth these days, however, there's definitely still work to be done. Men need to know that being overwhelmed by emotions is absolutely acceptable. If your heart gets broken, are you not a man if you cry? When you speak at your wedding and become emotionally overwhelmed, are you less of a man if you shed a tear? If your eyes get a little moist when you drop your daughter off at daycare for the first time, are you not acting in a manly way? The answer to these questions is an emphatic *no*. Without any doubt, you can still be a man *and* express your emotions. Forgive me for all the questions, but would you agree with me if I said that it's much healthier to *express* your emotions rather than *suppress* them for fear of not being manly? I have a feeling you would, and if you don't, just keep on reading. When all's said and done, emotionless equating manliness is a myth that needs to be broken apart

If anyone still needs convincing, let me tell you a bit more about the dangers of suppressing your emotions (because it's not "manly"). Being in denial about your emotions essentially means that you try to avoid expressing them, which, at best, is a very short-term solution. Ultimately, though, pushing your emotions away—or trying to avoid them on an ongoing basis—isn't going to do any favors for your mental health. It can lead to depression and anxiety, which is becoming more frequent, even as I write these words. As such, I would like to make it clear that there is a distinction between circumstantial depression and clinical depression. In life, we face trying circumstances like losing a loved one, being fired from our job, or being cheated on. I could list many more examples, but really, it comes down to sadness on a slightly lower level than just being a bit sad. Clinical depression is where you become so miserable to the point where you can't function for days on end. The point here is that not expressing your emotions is bad for your mental health, and also that men who experience anxiety should not be ashamed or feel like they are not... here we go again... "real men."

Successful Men Don't Meditate

By now, you're already aware that this is obviously untrue, thanks to our examples from earlier. But to take that discussion further, let's look at some more successful men who all practice meditation. Many of the following men attribute a significant part of their success to meditation.

- Bill Gates
  - As the computer engineer, author, philanthropist,

and billionaire who started Microsoft, Bill Gates is an avid fan of meditation.

- Michael Jordan
  - Arguably the best sportsman ever to play *any* sport, this basketball hero has been involved in business ventures that have been enormously successful, leading him to attain billionaire status.

- Mark Wahlberg
  - An actor of acclaim, Wahlberg has had a troubled past, including many run-ins with the law. But with age, he found meditation, and it changed his life for the better.

- Steve Jobs
  - Although Steve Jobs, the multibillionaire founder of Apple, succumbed to illness, he was outspoken about meditation's positive impact on his mental health.

- Arnold Schwarzenegger
  - Multiple Mr. Universe winner, movie star, and former Governor of California, Arnold Schwarzenegger has used meditation regularly ever since his days of fitness supremacy.

- Jeff Weiner
  - This venture capitalist and CEO of LinkedIn attributes meditation to his smart decision-making, emotional intelligence, and mental well-being enhancements.

- William Clay Ford Jr.
  - As a big exec at any massive company, there are challenges on a massive scale, and Ford Jr. has had his fair share. He combines mindfulness with meditation, deep breathing, and yoga to maintain mental alertness and strength during tough times. In fact, he says that, "The practice of mindfulness kept me going during the darkest days" (Natale & Welch, 2023).

If you weren't aware, the men above are among some of the most successful people in the world. Thus, I think a strong enough argument has been made against the myth that there are no successful males out there who meditate.

Meditation Is Really Just Doing Nothing

Of course it's not! Meditation is, in fact, doing a *lot* of things. Now, it's not doing a lot in the sense of moving around as if you were out jogging, or at the gym, but mentally, it can be highly intense. For one, the practice is more than just sitting down and making chanting noises. Meditation engages your brain, works on sensory observation, and as we saw in the previous chapter, has a plethora of benefits when it comes to mental *and* physical health. Breath control takes a lot of concentration, and concentration is a major workout for the brain. Taking all this into account, we can safely conclude that meditation is definitely *not* doing nothing. Though meditation can appear simple, when you fully immerse yourself in it, there's a lot of work you need to put in.

Breaking Barriers and Embracing Mindfulness

Meditation can be a barrier-breaker. And to a large extent, it is. Although men were the ones who pioneered meditation, there are barriers that exist, and we have touched on most—if not all of them—in this chapter and the previous one. However, meditation can do more than just break barriers; it can increase the quality of life in men who, before trying meditation, perhaps didn't ever expect to grow and feel fulfilled.

Now, I have managed to find a fantastic quote by a highly successful man, mentioned previously, which will serve for the purpose of motivation, and as a reminder that barriers have been broken, and will continue to be broken, starting with you, the reader:

> *No matter what you do, mindfulness is something that can get you ready for the moment, no matter how big or how small it is. Even if you're not trying to hit a game-winning shot in the NBA Finals, it's important to stay centered throughout any journey so that you can enjoy it all, and not just at the end of a big moment. Often, when people focus on the outcome instead of the process, they find themselves at the end asking, "Wow, is that it? And what now?" That's a difficult situation to be in. But if you're mindfully aware of all the moments up until that point, you won't get so stuck on what was or what could be. –Michael Jordan*

Indeed, Michael Jordan is an inspirational figure for millions of people worldwide, and his message on practicing meditation needs to reach as many individuals as possible. If it can work for one of the most successful men on the planet, it can *obviously* work for many more.

Chapter Takeaway

Reflecting on this chapter, we know that traditional definitions of manhood should be challenged, widened, changed, and altered. Debunking myths surrounding meditation is a good way to question and amend what it means to be "a real man." Meditation is not only for women; it was invented by men and is practiced by both sexes. Also, relying on meditation for your well-being is not a show of weakness and passivism—it's quite the opposite, as you've learned. Just taking up meditation means that you are strong enough to add positivity to your life. Furthermore, expressing emotions is far healthier than suppressing them, as the latter can lead to problems with anxiety and depression. We also look at a list of exceedingly successful men who rely on daily meditation, and the fact that they speak so highly of the practice is proof enough that it works. In closing, to be successful at what you do, you need forward momentum. And where does forward momentum come from? It comes from strength—which happens to be the subject of the next chapter.

CHAPTER 4:

Overcoming Stereotypes and Misconceptions - Embracing Meditation as a Man

—◆—

On one hand, I could say that it isn't necessary to discuss the relevance of meditation because by reading this book, you are giving it relevance. Nonetheless, I can guarantee that you're going to learn more about its relevance on a wider scale, mentally, physically, and otherwise. I should also mention that I've written another book, *Meditation for Beginners,* that is a bit more general and explains the various benefits and types of meditations on a wider scale. You may want to consider reading that as well. Here, though, we will now be looking at these same meditations as they specifically apply to *men*, and furthermore, how they can help men in their daily lives and challenges. Knowledge is indeed power, and to understand a concept, we have to harness knowledge.

> *The more man meditates upon good thoughts, the better will be his world and the world at large. —Confucius*

This message may sound obvious, but human beings have a strong leaning toward the negative, and the story I'm about to tell will show you just why that is.

Suppose you are in the great outdoors, and you see a snake in the grass. You are frightened, but also intrigued. You choose to investigate further, only to discover that what you thought was a snake is actually a belt. This story is part of an introduction to cognitive behavioral therapy, which you will learn about in chapters to come. The point, for now, is that the human brain *always* favors the worst scenario first. The good news, though, is that you can actually retrain your brain to favor the best or most positive outcome instead. If the outcome is good, then you haven't wasted any stress thinking about the worst-case scenario. And even if the outcome is a negative one, you still haven't wasted time on stress. I know, the latter statement might sound a bit strange, but think about it: Whether you were worried or not, the snake was either a snake or a belt, and thus the worry didn't change anything. This, then, means that there is no point in worrying! So, where do we go from here? Well, Confucius is highly respected in both Eastern and Western cultures, and as a result, his advocacy of meditation should be taken as coming from a *really* reliable source.

Now, in this chapter, we will be discussing what it means for men to become involved in daily mindful living on an ongoing basis. Self-forgiveness and forgiveness of others are more involved in meditation than you may think, and to that end, we'll also be looking at the transformative power that you can gain from meditation. From there, we'll go over some methods for handling stress on a daily basis, being emotionally resilient, and putting yourself in the best place possible to improve your cognitive function. Lastly, though memory and creativity form part of cognitive function, we can't discount physical and emotional well-being too. As such, we'll also cover that in this chapter, before finishing off with how to go about your first set of meditation exercises.

Shame as an Emotion

So many people feel shame—often unnecessarily. People with depression will often feel shame in one form and guilt in another.

Basically, shame is when we are assessing ourselves from another person's point of view. Meanwhile, guilt comes from our own judgment based on our own value system. If you're going through a particularly good time, you could very well feel guilt because you're not depressed during that period. It might sound strange, but this is actually regularly observed. A depressed person who's well placed in life, meaning they have a good job, a roof over their head, and enough food to eat, will feel guilt in the form of misplaced empathy toward people who don't require empathy. For instance, the guilt may be directed at another person who has an average job and doesn't make much money. The assumption—which is usually incorrect—is that this person must be unhappy because of their circumstances, when actually, they are perfectly happy and don't require much to live a fulfilling life. This is because they are living according to their own values, and not the values of someone else.

It's worth noting that men and women experience shame differently when it comes to the traits of masculinity and femininity. As we've discussed previously, males tend to be ashamed of parts of their personality or the ways that they act, which do not align with the societal definition of masculinity. If men aren't earning a lot of money and driving a fancy car, these are areas in which they can feel shame. Worst of all, this type of shame can manifest as anger or numbness. The former could be mixed in with jealousy of the apparent success of other males, while the latter could be a compartmentalization of the emotions associated with shame. Men are less expressive than women when it comes to shame, in that women are self-conscious about their appearance, and in recent times, content creators and social media influencers are to blame, because of the impossible standards they tend to set. As an antidote to shame, specifically, men likely have way more to get out of meditation than women.

Forgiveness

Shame can result from being wronged, usually by someone else, and not being able to let go of the negative emotions associated with that act of being wronged. If you are angry, frustrated, and resentful of someone who took advantage of you in some way, or embarrassed you in a public setting, then make no mistake— practicing forgiveness is the best method of getting rid of the negative feelings you have toward that other person.

Hate is far too powerful an emotion to waste on somebody
you really don't like.
–Unknown

There is so much truth to the above quote. Your attention is where you put your energy, and so, even when it comes to hate, you're bound to give too much power to the other person. At the same time, though, forgiveness is difficult to practice. However, in life, we need to face difficulties in order to progress and grow. So, to forgive, you need to make an internal decision to let go of any anger or resentment that you hold. Easier said than done? You bet, but remember that forgiving will improve your mental well-being, so you are actually doing it for yourself—not the other person. The positive effects of forgiveness are as follows:

- functional and healthy relationships
- better mental health
- reduced anxiety
- less aggression

The four points above are so positive that they're worth fighting for, especially when compared with the adverse effects of failing to forgive, as follows:

- dwelling on anger and bitterness to the point where you bring them into new relationships

- the inability to enjoy the present due to focusing on the past

- losing valuable connections with others

- irritability, anxiety, depression, or a combination of all three

So, you have the advantages of forgiveness and the disadvantages of holding grudges, but you need to know exactly *how* to forgive. Well, a good way to start making positive steps toward forgiveness is to write things down, and so I would encourage you to start keeping a journal. If you write, rather than type, then everything is visceral and more real. As an example, I will give you some points that you can write down, and spend time addressing:

- Accept that the incidents that have left you feeling wrong have happened, and cannot be changed.

- Be specific about the emotions that you feel, be they anger, hate, resentment, or others.

- Ask yourself whether being resentful is having a positive impact on your life. (Hint: it isn't!)

- Acknowledge that by failing to forgive, you are handing power over yourself to the other person.

- Come up with ways to forgive, and then put them into practice.

Sometimes, you can forgive someone, make amends, and move on, but if the person you intend to forgive is not interested in speaking to you again, you need to forgive them without actually communicating your forgiveness. Now, forgiveness doesn't always mean reconciliation, but if a rift has developed in a friendship or relationship that can be repaired by forgiveness *and* reconciliation, then I urge you to facilitate both. Either way, there are some positive affirmations or statements that you can write in your journal to help with the process. Let's take a look:

- *I have the capability to practice forgiveness.*

- *By forgiving, I am getting rid of a burden.*

- *One way to move forward and grow is through forgiveness.*

- *Everyone makes mistakes, and the person who hurt me made a mistake but deserves a second chance.*

- *Forgiveness will benefit me profoundly.*

Forgiveness also calls on vulnerability and evokes emotions, but remember that forgiving isn't a sign of weakness—it's a sign of strength. Holding a grudge never did anyone any good, and a saying that is often repeated when it comes to holding onto hurt is that "resentment is like drinking poison and hoping that your enemy dies" (Quote Investigator, 2017).

So, you may have done things that you regret, as has everyone else. And as a result, you may be carrying around some anger and resentment for yourself, thanks to the self-judgment you've engaged in, based on your personal value system. But guess what? The same logic applies to self-forgiveness. You have to acknowledge what you've done and accept that you've done it without casting judgment on yourself. Then, as explained above, you can truly practice forgiveness.

Of course, self-forgiveness is easier if the person you have wronged is available for an apology. Even if they don't accept the apology, though, you should still forgive yourself and take away any valuable lessons you can. When you do this, you allow yourself to learn from the mistakes you've made, and prevent yourself from making them going forward. Remember:

Forgiving heals the mind, body, and soul, as well as the course of your life.

Healing Practices

Be sure to check the references that follow the conclusion for a link to Alison Armstrong's fantastic approach to healing emotionally and mentally, specifically targeted at men, under the name "Noble Healing." You will find four videos that are absolutely free, and I certainly recommend watching them; you will learn a lot.

The Transformative Power of Meditation

Right, onto the main reason for reading this book. I wholeheartedly believe—from personal experience and observation of others—that meditation can change your life. The practice has certain elements, such as quieting the mind and then observing it in its quiet state, that are fundamental. In fact, our aim is to achieve these two fundamental elements in order to improve our mental and physical well-being.

Stress

We all experience stress, and even five minutes of meditation can act as a very helpful stress reliever. Stress reduction meditation comes in many forms, and I would like to give you some options.

- Breath meditation
  - You can do this exercise just about anywhere, but the best place to try it out for the first time is at home.
  - Sit in a comfortable chair with your back straight and

your feet on the ground, about shoulder-width apart.

○ When you are ready, close your eyes.

○ Take a deep breath in through your nose, and count to four as you feel your chest rising.

○ When you get to four, pause for a brief moment, and exhale through your mouth for another count of four.

○ Repeat for roughly five minutes.

○ Your aim is to focus on your breath and clear your mind of any thoughts. I can promise you that it will be difficult to maintain a clear mind at first, but when thoughts pop up, you need to acknowledge them, let them float away, and get back to focusing on your breathing.

○ You are basically distracting yourself from the worry and stress that you are experiencing. In fact, the very process of deep breathing brings your heart rate down, which promotes greater calm.

○ I said you can do this anywhere, and you can. However, if you are driving, sitting at your desk, or standing in a line at the grocery store, you will have to keep your eyes open!

- Affirmation meditation

○ This technique is also distraction-based and can be done anywhere. It's better to do it alone, though, because then you can speak out loud.

○ Get yourself into a comfortable position, either in a chair or lying down on your bed.

- Regulate your breathing without counting. Breathe normally, but a little bit slower than usual; your inhales and exhales should be the same length.

- While you breathe, recite affirmations in the form of solutions to the things you are stressed about (always in the present tense.) Suppose you have a big project at work, and you keep putting it off because it's so daunting. Here are some suggested affirmations that could be of use:

    - I am getting started, despite any difficulties.

    - I am *now* taking that step.

    - I am splitting up the project into smaller pieces and ticking them off as I go.

- The above are just suggestions, of course, and you can tailor your affirmations to suit yourself and your situation.

Emotional Resilience

We all find ourselves in times of trouble, when overwhelming situations lead to unpleasant emotions. It's difficult to stop those emotions, but they can be managed through a meditation practice specifically designed for emotional resilience.

- Exposure meditation
    - Instead of distracting yourself, this technique allows you to face your emotions and discover that they're not as bad as you may think.

    - Suppose you've recently been broken up with, and you're struggling to deal with the break up emotionally; this type of meditation can help.

- Again, choose a comfortable position, preferably with your eyes closed, and expose yourself to the situation that triggered your negative emotions. You can do so by visualizing the actual breakup.

- It will hurt, without a doubt, but the more you visualize, the more you trivialize, meaning that the event becomes less important, and thus, more conducive to emotional control.

- You can also visualize yourself doing well in the future, or engaging in activities that you find enjoyable. This is a way of proving to yourself that things aren't all that bad and that they *will* improve.

- 5-4-3-2-1

  - This type of meditation is also called "grounding," and you can see it as a way to bring yourself back down to earth, and out of your negative emotional state.

  - Keep your eyes open, and using your five senses, observe your immediate environment, noting the following:

    - five things you can see

    - four things you can feel

    - three things you can hear

    - two things you can smell

    - one thing you can taste

  - If you want to, you can run over the list a few times.

Try to really observe what you see, feel, hear, smell, and taste, in a way that makes you appreciate how incredible sensory engagement truly is.

Cognitive Improvement, Memory, and Clear Thinking

Meditation over an ongoing period can actually change the way your brain operates, improving cognitive function, as well as both focus and memory.

- Object focus

  - Get comfortable, regulate your breathing, and center yourself.

  - Have three objects in mind, and with your eyes closed, picture each object, one by one, without letting your mind stray. As I mentioned earlier, thoughts will pop up, but when they do, you can simply dismiss them and get back to the visualization.

  - Start with something simple, such as a stop sign. In your mind's eye, focus on the contrast in colors, the shape of the letters, the screws attaching the sign to the metal pole, etc.

  - By doing this, you are activating the four following areas in your brain:

    - the prefrontal cortex, which is charged with decision-making

    - the hippocampus, which is responsible for learning and memory

    - the gray matter, i.e., the part of your brain

that controls your senses, speech, and sight

- the amygdala, which is a part of your brain that regulates emotional responses

- Alphabet/name exercise
  - This exercise aims to engage your concentration, which helps with memory and clearer thinking.
  - Sit comfortably with your eyes closed, and regulate your breathing.
  - Recite the alphabet backward, i.e., Z, Y, X, and so on. It's not too easy to do, and that's precisely what I mean when I talk about concentration.
  - You could also go through the alphabet forward, and pick out one boy's name and one girl's name for each letter.
  - Either of the two options above will get your brain working, leading to an improvement in memory and clearer thinking.

Physical and Emotional Well-Being

Maintaining a balanced diet and making time in your day for some physical exercise are two excellent methods for maintaining physical well-being, which automatically leads to emotional well-being. Let's take a look at the importance of each, paying special attention to how lifestyle choices can influence day-to-day living, both positively and negatively.

Physical Well-Being

I don't have to tell you, but hey, I'm going to anyway: Smoking and excessive alcohol consumption do nothing good for your health, and hence, they negatively impact your physical well-being. You know these things, and if you're prone to cigarettes and liquor, you should try to give them up, or at the very least, cut down as much as possible. We all have busy lives, but you can definitely find 30 minutes, four days a week to exercise. If you're not currently doing any physical activity, start with a half-hour walk every other day, and after a month to six weeks, you'll observe a change in your fitness level. Indeed, you'll feel good physically, and thanks to this feeling, you'll also feel good *mentally*. Next, you have to think about your eating habits. It's so easy to have anything delivered to your door these days, and that means that you can have healthy meals delivered—or just ingredients for healthy meals. Think balance and moderation, and you will start feeling better physically, with a clearer and more alert mind.

Emotional Well-Being

As you now know, our physical and mental well-being are tied together in so many ways. If you can manage your emotions through meditation—and you *can*—then life can be more fulfilling. Hobbies help with emotional well-being, as they engage your mind, and in many cases, also your body. Perhaps you like yoga or playing a musical instrument. Maybe you would like to learn how to play a musical instrument or join a debating society. The point is, increasing the amount of hobbies you have fills your time, and instead of stressing, worrying, or experiencing anxiety, you're engaging in something positive. Hobbies also allow you to draw fulfillment from life, and in times when you aren't satisfied in other areas, like work or romantic relationships, fulfillment can come from your hobbies. Feeling unfulfilled is a pretty awful feeling, and is, of course, associated with negativity, meaning that fulfillment is your path to positivity. You can strive for fulfillment at work, in your relationships, or in any area of your life for that matter. Regardless, what you do in your free time can act as a major emotional boost. So, if you already have hobbies, keep doing them, and if you don't, find some!

Creating Healthy Connections

Have you ever had such a bad day that when you stubbed your toe on the coffee table by mistake, you blamed the table? We all have, and we can all empathize, but the negative connections that you associate with what happened during your day are what cause the peak of your anger, despair, or frustration. With that in mind, we need to make positive associations as much as we can, and part of that involves picking yourself up after something negative happens and telling yourself to *keep going*. With every mistake, you should connect a chance to learn and to do things differently the next time around. Let's take something that may seem insignificant to you—having a tidy bedroom. Making your bed in the morning, having neatly folded clothes in your dresser, and getting rid of clutter all provide a safe space. When you walk into your room, you should associate it with calm, and you should make that same association on an ongoing basis in all situations. Toxic friendships or dysfunctional relations create negative associations, meaning that you connect them with negativity. If you suspect you may be in a toxic friendship or dysfunctional relationship, take time to ask yourself if you need the negativity that connects you with that connection, and if not, leave it for a healthier one. You need to set your sights on quality time, shared activities, and emotional intimacy.

Meditation Exercises for Physical and Emotional Well-Being

The interconnectedness of the physical and the mental is clear, and there are certainly several types of meditation, including mindfulness that target both. Let's have a look at them.

Diaphragmatic Breathing

This technique is also known as "belly breathing," and as the two names suggest, you need to draw air in through your nose and into your belly, hold briefly, and release. You can sit or lie down for this, preferably the latter, and use the four-count method. Simply breathe in deeply through your nose while you count to four, and observe your belly filling up with air. Then, after a brief pause, exhale deeply, also counting to four along the way. The idea is to focus only on your breath and have your mind clear. You know what to do when stray thoughts pop up— acknowledge them, and let them float away.

The Mindful Body Scan

Sit comfortably in a chair with your hands in your lap, or lie down on your back with your hands at your sides. You can breathe as you normally would for this one. In your mind's eye, picture your toes, and notice how they feel when you wiggle them. Move onto your shins, and observe the energy around them. Head up to your quads—picture them and the specific detail they have. Carry on until you reach the top of your head, and then make your way back down to your toes. There is no prescribed time period for this, just don't rush. Take as long as you like, and refocus when you need to.

Loving Kindness Meditation

It's always good to be *loving* and to show *kindness*, but both can be a challenge at times. Thankfully, there's a meditation with these exact feelings in mind! Convincing your brain that you're loving and kind will connect with genuinely being loving and kind. Again, get comfortable, and like the body scan, breathe normally. If you're feeling worried or anxious, then it's best to regulate your breathing before you start. Then, all you have to do is recite some statements. Saying them out loud is best, and after you have finished your meditation session, you can write them down. Now, here are a few examples:

- I can and will give love and be kind to people.

- In return, I deserve love and kindness.

- Loving others and being kind to them will make them love me in return, and be kind to me as well.

Then, you can think of some people you should be treating well, and recite some statements directed at them. These could include the following:

- I want you to be physically and mentally healthy.

- You deserve love and kindness.

- You are unique and worthy of love.

Feel free to get creative and come up with your own statements.

Guided Visualization

This takes the object focus method a bit further, and is often done in conjunction with a therapist, who will guide you through visualization exercises. However, a therapist isn't essential, and you can access guided visualization meditations on Spotify, Apple Music, YouTube, or any other music/content-sharing platform. Perhaps you want to visualize your perfect day, a beach scene, or a walk in the mountains. Whatever you choose, the goal is to remain in that state of visualization for as long as possible. By doing this, your brain is going through something pleasurable in a virtual sense. The more you practice this exercise, the deeper you can get into the scenes you visualize, and the clearer your mind will become.

Chapter Takeaway

Shame is an unpleasant emotion, and so is guilt, as we've covered in this chapter. Meanwhile, we learned that stress, emotional resilience, cognitive function, memory, and clear thinking make up the transformative power of meditation. Indeed, you now have instructions on the most relevant types of meditation that work best in each of the categories discussed. From a physical perspective, try to change your diet and any bad habits if you need to. Also, introduce exercise into your life, and always strive for positive connections, whether they have to do with people or behaviors. Finally, we looked at some types of meditation that can assist in promoting good physical and emotional health, so keeping those in mind, let's now press on to address how you can truly embrace meditation as a man.

CHAPTER 5:

Unleashing Masculine Energy - Meditation for Personal Growth

—◆—

To know yourself is to be confident.
To be confident is to fearlessly express your potential.
—Andy Puddicombe

For those of you who don't know, Andy Puddicombe is a British author, public speaker, and staunch advocate of meditation and mindfulness. We could add to his quote above and say that growth into yourself and who you really want to be are also steps in the process of fearless expression of self. Regardless, with his words in mind, this chapter is going to find us applying meditation as a way to unleash masculine energy for the purpose of both personal growth and development.

What Is Masculine Energy?

Of course, before you unleash masculine energy, you need to know what it *is*. An important point to note is that many women also have masculine energy, just not as much as men, and vice versa. That said, male energy is most often action-oriented and relatively predictable, while female energy is less predictable and more fluid. Both are good types of energy, though, and that's why we want to use our masculine energy to *grow*. Now, I'd like to make the picture clearer by setting out traits of masculine energy, followed by trains of feminine energy. Don't forget that this topic is a complex one, and as such, there are a number of books dedicated specifically to it. I mention this to confirm that we'll just be looking at a summary right now, and so if you wish to expand your knowledge, then please do so through additional resources.

- Masculine
  - enjoys taking on challenges
  - thrives in competition
  - has good problem-solving skills and creativity
  - seeks out the point of the problem that requires solving
  - has a proclivity to "single focus," which is when everything but the point of focus is pushed into the background, and becomes a figurative blur
  - has a strong sense of independence
  - wants to feel appreciated
  - thinks rationally and logically
  - is externally strong
  - has the ability to see things through to their conclusion
- Feminine
  - has the ability to empathize
  - requires communication in order to connect
  - practices self-care and self-love
  - has a good relationship with emotions, i.e.,

recognizes them more easily and releases them
appropriately

- ○ looks for creative inspiration
- ○ prioritizes feelings

As you can tell, these are all—or mostly are—good parts of one's
energy, and there are mostly complementary characteristics. But
for now, of course, we are focused on the masculine energy side.
Again, this is a summary, and I would encourage you to explore
other literature on this specific topic.

Something we have to consider is the brain/body connection,
because it's present when you're using your energy negatively,
and it's also present when you're using your energy in a positive
way. Meditation, although not physically demanding, falls into
the positive category. Besides that, masculine energy fuels the
need to take on challenges, solve problems, and see things
through to their conclusion. Just by choosing to take on
meditation, you are pushing your masculine energy toward a
practice that will provide a release—and a wonderful outlet, at
that. All the traits you have, regarding seeing something through,
need to come to the surface, and your commitment will be
rewarded.

Masculine energy directs and essentially says what needs to
happen, however, this cannot be done without the creative
feminine energy, which we also all carry with us. See, it's mostly
a stereotype that the man is the one with 100% masculine energy,
and the woman with 100% feminine energy. In reality, it can
actually be more complex than that, and the objective is that we
all have both energies working within while presenting the
dominant one to create our reality. In this case, meditation is a
powerful tool to change gears.

Creating Synergy

We talked about this briefly in the Introduction, but let's expand on this now. To put it plainly, synergy is the combined power of a group of things when they are working *together*, which is greater than the total power achieved by each working *separately* (Cambridge Dictionary, n.d.). That's synergy. Now, synergy is one of those words that you just know when to use, without thinking of the mechanics of what it means. That's my experience, anyway. It's often used in sports when referring to a team who are in tune with each other, working together in equal parts to create a dominant force—*synergy*. It's also used in the workplace when the employees are all pulling in the same direction. However, for our purposes here, synergy will be used in the context of—you guessed it—meditation. But, what is the "group of things" in this case? Well, when it comes to meditation, it's a minimum of two things: the body and the mind. Indeed, when working together, you have a synergy that makes you the best version of yourself.

And it's not only about the external or even the internal. When practiced by a number of people, it can improve one's social environment. This idea is defined as the "Maharishi Effect," which I detailed in my previous book.

The influence of coherence and positivity in the social and natural environment is generated by the practice of Transcendental Meditation (Maharishi International University, n.d.).

How to Use Meditation and Mindfulness to Support Your Physical Health

You may remember the mindful body scan we talked about back in Chapter 3, but there are several more techniques that we can learn when it comes to mindfulness. Presence and focus are associated with both mindfulness and meditation and, as you are aware, there are several crossovers. Mindfulness is a practice that can be employed before, during, and after meditation sessions. And due to its success, I would be remiss if I didn't explain both. After all, the more you know about mindfulness, the more you can use it for positive results.

Mindful Eating

Because of the fast pace of life, we often wolf down our lunch, drop the plate, and keep on working. But when we do this, we don't take time to enjoy it. We don't focus on each bite. When you practice mindful eating, though, you're trying to be present in the moments of biting, chewing, and swallowing. Chances are you usually check your phone between mouthfuls; many of us do. However, that rush, with your mind on what's coming next, takes you out of the moment. So, put down your phone, close your laptop, and appreciate the food. Draw distinctions between the colors of herbs, vegetables, meat, and whatever else is on your plate. Then, take your first bite, chew slowly, and pay attention to the texture, as your teeth break it up, and then the tastes as they mix together. Observe the feeling as your first bite goes down your throat, and then repeat the process. If your mind wanders, bring it back to the eating experience, and refocus on enjoying the tastes of the moment. In rudimentary terms, you are giving yourself a break from the stress, worry, and, of course, phone obsession.

Mindful Commuting

Commuting is an inconvenience that's difficult to avoid. It can even be a stress-inducer. So, if you drive to work, look around for things to occupy your mind—whether that's the bright red car in the lane next to you, the trees blowing in the wind, or the people walking past. You will appreciate how interesting seemingly mundane sights and sounds can be when you observe the little details. This deep focus on what surrounds you allows you to stay in the present, and enjoy it as much as possible, without thinking of yesterday or tomorrow. If you walk to work, you have a great opportunity to look around and enjoy your surroundings. Listen carefully to the birds, the traffic, or both. Even though the sound of traffic isn't a great one, it helps to pick out specific sounds, within the overall hum, which takes the kind of concentration that keeps your mind relatively free of thought.

The two examples above make the aim clear, and you can apply these methods to cooking, grocery shopping, and basically any situation where you have surroundings to observe.

Gratitude Walk/Run

Exercise is always recommended, and if you can get the physical benefit from walking or running, you might as well get the mental benefit too. The idea is to think of and focus on all the things you're grateful for. In fact, you'll probably be surprised at how many things are on your gratitude list. It might seem obvious, but I'm sure you're grateful for the sun, and that you have a roof over your head. So, while you run or walk, focus on how fortunate you are. You might also be grateful for having a job, even though the job may not be what you thought it would be when you started it. There will be people in your life you're grateful for, too, and those will likely consist of family, friends, colleagues, and even bosses, depending on your situation. Think of absolutely *everything*, because with each grateful thought comes positivity, and distraction from harmful and/or negative thinking.

Journaling

We've also discussed this previously, but I must bring it up again—for good reason. Besides being a way to chronicle your life, keeping a journal partially dedicated to mindfulness practices will serve you well. This book is part of a Meditation Series, and you can check out the meditation journal that comes with this book, as well as other resources such as coloring books. You can use your discretion when it comes to what you write, but gratitude is obviously a great idea, as well as positive affirmations. We can trick our brains into erring on the side of positivity, although it's more natural to head toward the negative as your first reaction; we're just designed that way, unfortunately. Now, cognitive behavioral therapy (CBT), which is closely related to mindfulness, can offer us a very good example. Suppose your phone rings, and it's someone who never calls. Your immediate thought is that it must be bad news, but really, that person is just calling for a catch-up since they haven't made contact with you in a long time. Positive affirmations in your journal are also an excellent method to favor positivity over negativity. You can then carry this over into actual life situations. Recording your progress in your diary is also a means to improve, work on yourself, and grow. With this purpose, I created a meditation journal https://mybook.to/meditation_workbook, which is part of the series.

Self-Discovery

Many people go through life without understanding themselves, and that's honestly understandable, considering how complicated human beings are. However, if you can *really* understand yourself, you can become comfortable with yourself as a whole, and from there, create the best version of yourself on an ongoing basis. In order to discover yourself, though, you need to sit down with a pen in hand and list all the good parts, as well as all the bad parts. You can't love everything about yourself, and that's okay, but the aim of this exercise is acceptance *without judgment*. When you have everything, and I mean everything—

including regrets or ways that you could have acted differently in the past—then you can write about successes you've enjoyed, reasons why your friends and family love you, as well as any good you've done to change the lives of others. Knowledge is power, and when you have knowledge in the form of written evidence, believe me, you can work on improving your weak points while maintaining your good points. Now, let's take a look at some more tips for self-discovery and self-growth:

- Work on being your best self all the time, and not only when you're around other people. Implement small things, like keeping your home tidy, making your bed in the morning, and removing clutter, so you're in a positive environment.

- Take your strengths and apply them in a bigger way than you are currently. If you can use your strengths to help other people, then even better.

- Ask lots of questions and learn from others, especially individuals who are older than you and have more life experience.

- Start building good habits that develop into a positive daily routine.

- Get out of your comfort zone. Sometimes we need to get uncomfortable to get comfortable.

- Find the things you're passionate about, and spend time on those things, whatever they may be.

- Surround yourself with the right people, as in the ones who love you and want the best for you, as opposed to those who bring you down.

- It's such a cliché, but like most clichés, it's true, so I will say it: Learn from your mistakes. Try to avoid them, of course, but when you make them, take stock without self-judgment, remedy the situation if possible, and act differently in the future. I'm not saying that you get a free pass to make mistakes, but you know what I mean when I talk about *non-self-judgment.*

When it comes to breaking down the myth that men shouldn't be introspective, there's something we should engage with—and that's self-discovery. . To be blunt, if you can't manage this, you won't be able to benefit from most of the tips, techniques, advice, and explanations in this book. Ask yourself—would you rather know yourself, feel fulfilled, and be seen as less of a man, or unsure of yourself, unfulfilled, but viewed as a real man? I think I know the answer!

Vulnerability

Allowing yourself to be vulnerable is a sign of strength—not of weakness. Why? Because you're putting yourself out there, taking risks, and exposing yourself to the unknown; a formula for growth. Also included in the wider context of vulnerability is *self-awareness.* Vulnerability is incredibly hard to show, or even to allow yourself to feel, as it can be painful to acknowledge your mistakes, anxieties, or fears. So, don't discount the fact that being vulnerable has the potential to impact other people and your relationships with them.

> *Self-awareness is your ability to perceive and understand the things that make you who you are as an individual, including your personality, actions, values, beliefs, emotions, and thoughts. Essentially, it is a psychological state in which the self becomes the focus of attention. —Kendra Cherry*

There's a close relationship between self-discovery and self-awareness, but one could argue that you need to discover the real you in order to become self-aware. Some people feel that the opposite is true, but either way, the two inform each other.

Public Self-Awareness

When you're out in public, it's almost impossible to be the exact same person you are when you're alone or with close friends or family. If eyes are on you, you may want to act appropriately and be your best self, which is something you should also be doing when you're not in the social spotlight. We can include the workplace as a public setting in which you're self-aware, in that you don't want to do or say something inappropriate that may cause issues. Having said that, you still need to be true to yourself, and not let others cross your boundaries or take advantage of you. The bottom line is that none of us are constant, and our self-awareness is always changing.

Private Self-Awareness

This could be as simple as looking at yourself in the mirror, which is a manner of being self-aware when you're on your own. On top of that, try to consider the fact that your guard is dropped when you're alone, including when you're spending time with the people whom you value the most. You can be yourself—and you *should* be yourself at all times—even though your private and public selves may differ. Believe me, you're not alone in embracing self-awareness differently in different situations.

The Elements of Self-Awareness

We can break the concept down into further categories that form a logical path, ending with self-awareness as a whole. Let's take a closer look:

- Consciousness
  - The fact that you are alive and thinking means that you are conscious. Furthermore, you're aware of your emotions, thoughts, and feelings, which is further proof that your cognition is, well, operational.
- Emotional intelligence
  - We spoke about this earlier, and again, it comes down to the way you deal with other people, understanding and managing emotions on both sides.
- Self-acceptance
  - Remember how, when we discussed self-discovery earlier, I said that you need to accept the good and the bad? Well, the exact same scenario is at play when it comes to self-acceptance.
- Self-knowledge
  - Ask yourself what your beliefs, values, and motivation sources are in order to create more knowledge about yourself.
- Self-reflection
  - This is the ability to be introspective. Furthermore, it's the ability to think deeply about your feelings and emotions and develop an understanding of where you are in life, along with where you want to be.

Meditation, because of its introspective nature, can help you find your self-awareness, and at the same time become comfortable with yourself in a wider sense.

Emotional Resilience Through Meditation

There are many times in life when we need to be resilient; some are big and others are not so big. Losing a loved one or going through a messy divorce calls for emotional resilience, as do receiving a poor performance review at work or failing to keep up with your fitness regime. Because of the alignment of body and mind, meditation can be of great assistance in difficult times, during which you definitely have to be resilient. To understand this, we need to break down what resilience actually is. Take a look:

- Emotional regulation
  - One key part of resilience is the ability to manage your emotions in times of stress and distress. This must not be confused with emotional suppression, as we know how bad that can be for one's mental well-being. Rather, it's a case of feeling the emotions and accepting them for what they are, but also exercising control over them.

- The survivor mentality
  - Believing and really *knowing* that you can get through whatever's thrown your way can demonstrate that you're a survivor and not just a passenger.

- Problem-solving skills
  - When we face problems, it can sometimes seem like solutions are far off. In these cases, a calm disposition and a willingness to explore every possible solution can give you a foot up when it comes to finding the right solution.

- Self-compassion
  - Where an opportunity presents itself, you need to be kind to yourself. Indeed, when you think of the kind of compassion you show to others, you should be applying the same kind of compassion to yourself.
- A solid support system
  - Without support, it's difficult to be resilient. And without a doubt, every single one of us has weak moments where we need to call on someone in our support network to give us that pep talk and prop us back up.

All I can say is... When times get tough, meditate.

Strength and Clarity

I'm not talking about physical strength here, but rather, *mental* strength. When you start becoming mentally strong, you gain a different perspective, and most often it's a clearer one. If you're also physically fit, your mind is just about automatically in tune with your body, which actually makes your power of concentration longer when it comes to meditation sessions. This is because meditation—when combined with mindfulness—is a way to soothe your mind. It's like clearing clutter off a shelf and replacing it with something valuable. In a human sense, that value is in the form of clearer thought—and we already know the decision-making benefits of clarity.

When Challenges Become Opportunities

I didn't fail 1,000 times. The light bulb was an invention with

1,000 steps. –Thomas Edison

Just about everyone knows Thomas Edison as the inventor of the lightbulb, but I bet you didn't know that the road to light was a long one, as illustrated by his quote above; no doubt a great way to look at a challenge.

Some of us become overwhelmed in the face of a challenge, but remember, if you direct your masculine energy to the right places, you can channel that energy to give yourself the strength to take on challenges, as well as to succeed in achieving what it is that you want. Mastering meditation—and it may be the case that nobody has absolutely, positively mastered it—is a challenge in itself. Luckily, though, there's a simple approach you can take when accepting the challenge to master meditation, and it comes in the form of an acronym: S.M.A.R.T. Remember this from the Introduction? Well, now we're *really* going to explore it. First of all, this acronym actually represents goal setting in a stripped-down way. It incorporates **s**pecific, **m**easurable, **a**chievable, **r**elevant, and **t**ime-bound goals; let me explain further.

- **S**pecific
  - If you say your goal is to lose weight, that's quite broad. However, you can make it more specific by putting a *number* to it. So, you may want to lose *seven* pounds or cut your waistline by *three* inches. This is also ambiguous, though, because first, you need to gain the weight and then lose it. As you can tell, the words we use are extremely important. So, the goal is "getting to your desired weight and achieving your ideal waistline." When it comes to meditation, your goal could be to do a breathing exercise for five minutes without a thought entering your mind.

- **M**easurable

  - Regarding weight loss, the goal is obviously measurable, because you can keep track of both your weight and your waistline. In terms of the meditation example, though, it's a little more complicated because you don't really want to stop midway when your first thought pops up. However, by sneaking a quick glance at your watch as you dismiss the thought, you can give yourself time to return to your meditative state, void of thoughts.

- **A**chievable

  - Losing 50 pounds is probably not achievable, but if it is, then you're thinking long-term. However, you can have some interim checkpoints, at say five, seven, or ten pounds. Meditation-wise, five minutes is definitely achievable, and when you get there, you can set another specific goal to pursue.

- **R**elevant

  - In the meditation case, achieving five minutes without thought is relevant.

- **T**ime-bound

  - If you don't set a time period, your goal will become less specific. You may want to shed the pounds and shrink the waistline within six months, and the same time period could apply to meditation... Well, it's up to you, but just be realistic. The point is, you need to mention these goals through affirmations every day, which is also time-related, of course.

Other challenges you can apply the S.M.A.R.T. framework to may be achieving a promotion at work, getting an A on an assignment at school, scoring five goals over the course of your soccer season, or reaching certain landmarks when learning a musical instrument. Whatever the challenge, you have a standard set of guidelines to follow, which will allow you to truly fulfill the opportunities you create.

Chapter Takeaway

As Andy Puddicombe reminded us at the onset of this chapter, to be confident is to fearlessly express your potential. To do this, you have your masculine energy to call on but don't forget that you also have a small amount of valuable feminine energy too. Use your mind and body connection to create synergy, and involve yourself in mindfulness to accentuate it. We've also talked about journaling, and how it can help you in the pursuit of self-discovery. Don't forget to identify your strengths, weaknesses, and everything else about you for the purposes of acceptance and growth. From there, develop good habits, follow your passions, and meditate! On top of that, take advantage of the S.M.A.R.T. goal-setting framework, as you can apply it in all areas of your life. Lastly, something that you should always consider is remaining *authentic*, and guess what? That's going to be the centerpiece of our next chapter! So, please join me as we now move on to discussing all things authenticity and its relationship with meditation.

CHAPTER 6:

Empowering Men Through Meditation - Embracing Authenticity

—◆—

The ultimate measure of a man is not where he stands in moments of comfort and convenience but where he stands at times of challenge and controversy. –Martin Luther King Jr.

If you go through life and never experience what it's like to be uncomfortable, then I'm sorry to say, but you're bound to stunt your personal growth. Now, if there was ever a man who faced seemingly insurmountable challenges, and involved himself in necessary controversy, that man was Martin Luther King Jr. Some people are born to challenge the status quo, no matter how small it may seem in the "bigger picture." If you can stand up when things are just not right and have a voice, then you're certainly empowering yourself, and showing authenticity where others have failed to do so. Being authentic is hard work, of course, and that's the reason why there's so little authenticity in life. Yes, society imposes expectations, but we have the power to live up to our own expectations, and not the imposed expectations. And now, as we progress through this chapter, you're going to learn all about how meditation can create a more authentic and fuller life for yourself.

The Power of Authenticity

The ability to be your absolute authentic self can be both a blessing and a curse. It's a blessing because it's admirable to be yourself, and thus not adhere to what society expects, but it's a curse because individuality and authenticity can be pretty poorly received as a result of those expectations. Now, depending on where you are, there's still a certain amount of homophobia, but back in the 1980s, coming out as gay and being your authentic self was met with disapproval, hate, and violence. Thankfully, we have progressed, and trust me—embracing meditation to assist in your ongoing authenticity is the right course of action. Manliness—whatever that is—comes back into the conversation here, as many men hold back on their emotions, as we've discussed, and may also alter their disposition in order to appear "manly." When you start meditating, it will become part of your authentic self, and hiding it because you're concerned with others speculating about you being a real man will do you no good—plain and simple. This applies across the board, and as such, you should strive to be *you* as much as possible, and as often as you can. If you fear judgment, try to remember that this fear only makes you human, and you can lessen it by exposing yourself to criticism.

Mindful Self-Compassion

This term is definable as follows:

Mindful self-compassion (MSC) is the process of combining the skills developed through mindfulness with the emotional practice of self-compassion (Mead, 2019).

Usually, we're capable of showing more compassion to others than ourselves, and more often than not, we're also our own harshest critics. If a person accidentally says something offensive to their friend, you would likely tell that person not to beat themselves up about it, but rather to apologize and make amends. Furthermore, you'd explain to your friends that it's not as bad as they are making it out to be, and they shouldn't be so hard on themselves. However, it's likely that you don't show the same compassion to yourself when you're the one who's made a mistake. As Mead's definition points out, you are looking to combine mindfulness with self-compassion in order to get some synergy firing.

By turning compassion inward, you can work on your emotional development, including your ability to *accept*. Mindfulness is about paying attention to the whole experience, be it mundane or interesting. When we add self-compassion, we can see that it's generally founded on the principle of accepting negative experiences or emotions without judgment. Fortunately, mindful self-compassion can be learned, and in many situations, it should be practiced much more frequently. There are many ways to be mindfully self-compassionate, and with a little bit of practice, it will come easily. Let's explore some of those ways right now:

- Self-kindness
  - Accepting your mistakes is an aspect of self-kindness in that you need to forgive yourself in order to move forward, but it goes further than that.
  - You want to have a positive self-image, and by placing focus on your strengths, you can do just that.
  - Journaling is useful in this regard, as it is in so many, and so an idea here is to write down or type out some positive statements about yourself and put them in areas of your home where you can regularly see them (next to your bed, on the fridge, etc.). Get creative!
  - Treat yourself to things that you enjoy. This could

include a massage, going for a walk, watching TV all day, getting into a good book, or learning something new.

- Common humanity

  - Caring for our fellow humans is something we should all embrace more. You can do the smallest things, like saying hello to an elderly man or complimenting the teller at the grocery store on how good her hair looks, and these will spread kindness. And it flows both ways!

  - If you can be compassionate to a stranger—and we all should—then you can definitely be compassionate to yourself.

- Reframing personal criticism

  - If you're particularly hard on yourself in some areas, then you're probably being overly critical, and the reality is that the situation is likely not as bad as you're making it out to be. These are some questions you can ask yourself that will lead to the act of reframing I'm talking about:

    - Am I still myself when I show this trait?

    - How often do I display this trait?

    - Is it circumstantial, or is it something I do in different scenarios?

    - Do I have a choice, or is the trait automatic?

    - How can I reframe my thoughts about this trait?

  - Suppose you're easily irritated, and your interactions

with colleagues at work bring this out. Basically, when something is done in a way that's different from what you would do if the task was yours, you show your irritation toward the colleague responsible.

○ By knowing the circumstances, you can reframe your approach. You have to set your expectations in a way that you accept different ways of doing things. When mistakes happen, it's best to acknowledge them and explain to your colleague what the error is, as well as how to rectify it. You should remain calm because you *know* that we all do things in different ways.

○ Tell yourself that you have a choice—which is true—and make an effort to use the approach discussed above.

○ Don't be too self-critical about your trait, and remember to use reframed language. So, instead of saying, "I always get irritated when X, Y, or Z happens," say, "Sometimes I get irritated when X, Y, or Z happens."

○ At this stage, you will slowly realize that you can address concerns while remaining calm, and furthermore, you can treat other people the way you would like to be treated. Soon, your "sometimes" will turn into "seldom" and then "almost never." It's impossible to go through life without irritation, so "never" is unrealistic.

○ As your levels of irritation lessen, you will have less to criticize yourself about, and that opens the door to self-compassion, especially when you notice you've done the work and that things are moving in a positive direction.

Self-Reflection

The benefits of self-reflection are vast, and doing acts of self-reflection regularly paves the road to better self-understanding. Of course, meditation and mindfulness play a role too, self-reflection exercises on their own are certainly great options. Having said that, I would always recommend employing mindfulness whenever you can. Now, let's start with the benefits:

- A deeper sense of control

  - Being present is a way to exercise control over your emotions (not repressing them) and actions, which create a clearer picture and make decision-making more effective.

- Better communication skills

  - If you understand what you're feeling, you can express yourself better, which is a big help when it comes to maintaining healthy relationships in all contexts.

- Self-awareness

  - When you gain a deeper knowledge of your emotions, thoughts, and behaviors through self-reflection, you can enhance your emotional intelligence, and thus interact with other people in a kind and compassionate manner.

- Looking after core values

  - Oftentimes, we're not specific enough about our

morals, values, and boundaries. This results in people having an easier time taking advantage of us, and crossing our boundaries. After all, if your boundaries are vague or not communicated, other people have no way of knowing if they're crossing them.

- Accountability
  - Not accepting responsibility when you should is not going to help you in any way. It's a bit like emotional suppression, and the mental well-being impact can be profound. If you've fumbled in some way, you need to accept this and implement changes to remedy the situation.

There can be a fine line between positive and negative self-reflection, but as you now know, reframing negative thoughts is what you're aiming for. For the sake of completeness, I would now like to set out what *not to do* when it comes to self-reflection.

- Self-judgment
  - This is what we're trying to avoid, as judging yourself negatively in any context is definitely not the way to go about productive self-reflection.

- Rumination
  - Rather than dwell on the bad points and run them over and over in your head, you need to acknowledge and address them. So, instead of thinking, "I should have done this differently, " think, "Next time, I will do this differently." You can then move forward instead of being stuck in a negative loop.

- Negative self-talk
  - This can be reduced to anything simple that you complain about, even if you're complaining internally. Yes, going to the grocery store is a chore, but try not to see it like that. Make your trip a mindful one, as you observe the sights, sounds, smells, and everything else associated from the time you leave the house to the time you return.

- Comparison
  - This can send you into another negativity loop. Comparing yourself to others is not going to be productive by any stretch of the imagination.

  - As an unrelated example, in terms of the subject, I would like to set out a situation in which comparing yourself *today* to yourself *yesterday* works. So, let's say you decide to train for a 10-mile race. You have a time goal, and after every training run, you record your time so that you can compare your time today to your time yesterday, and thus track your progress.

  - In the above example, you aren't going to be comparing your times to the times of elite athletes. That would only lead to disappointment, obviously, so whatever you do, don't compare yourself to others when you're self-reflecting. Measure your progress against yourself and *only* yourself!

With the above in mind, here are some tips to help you get going with self-reflection:

- Always use open questions.

- Am I taking anything for granted in my life? If I am, what is it, and how can I change it?

- What repetitive thoughts am I having? Are they positive or negative? If they're negative, how can I reframe them?

- Am I being kind to myself, and doing the things that make me happy?

  - If you are, that's fantastic, and you have the right to congratulate yourself.

  - If you're not, then you can come up with some options to do what it is that will make you happy.

- Process your emotions.

  - Think of things that happened during your day, or the day before, and allow yourself to feel the emotions, whether good or bad. Then, decide what to do with those emotions—either let them go or change them.

  - By now, you're probably aware of how big on journaling I am, but really, this is another great opportunity to use your journal to process your emotions.

- Create a positive self-reflection board.

  - It doesn't have to be a board, per se. As long as it's something that you can add positive affirmations to, or methods to stay true to yourself and record the things that you're doing well, then you're on the right track.

In general, always make sure you have at least 30 minutes for self-reflection, as this is something you definitely don't want to rush. You may want to make it part of your daily routine, in fact, or perhaps do it every other day. Take caution, though, as it's something you can easily let slide. So, make a conscious effort to self-reflect regularly, and your quality of mental health will, without a doubt, improve. Also, always choose a quiet area for this—one free from distractions, and without the possibility of being interrupted.

Communication

Alright, we've touched briefly on improved communication skills, and now it's time to expand further. It may sound obvious, but men and women communicate in different ways, with each other *and* with the opposite sex. As such, we need to understand these different types of communication in order to gain knowledge of our communication style, and how to improve it where necessary.

Male Versus Female Communication

- Men tend to build friendships on a side-by-side basis and maintain that friendship through shared activities. Women, in contrast, have a more face-to-face way of cultivating friendships. As a very general example, men may bond over sports, while women may bond over coffee or lunch dates.

- For men, there is less intimacy involved—not physically, but in terms of not getting too deep when discussing emotions. Women, on the other hand, are far more likely to open up to each other and talk about their emotions, feelings, thoughts, and experiences.

- After an argument, men are much more likely to remain friends, as opposed to women, who may fall out permanently, or for an elongated period.

- Men will consider someone as a friend even if they have irregular contact. Women, though, prefer to be in more constant contact so that they can grow the friendship.

- Women often have quite fragile relationships, meaning that it's easier to upset the other person emotionally, while men usually build stronger relationships, possibly because of the intimacy distance.

- Men tend to hang out in groups, whereas women favor one-on-one interactions.

- Men, more often than women, use sarcasm and good-natured taunts, which women might see as offensive if they were to do the same thing with their friends.

Authentic Communication

Have you ever had a friendship where you needed to tone yourself down or act in a way that didn't truly reflect your authenticity? I think most people have, and perhaps you've experienced a type of friendship where your interests didn't quite align, and so you adapted your actions to create a false alignment. You may have felt bad for the other person because you were their only friend, even though they were taking way more out of the friendship than you are. This is quite a delicate situation because, obviously, you *want* to be yourself, but by being yourself, you may hurt the other person. Ultimately, though, pretending you have the same interests or opinions isn't going to do any good for either party. I realize that these can be tricky situations, but if you're in one right now, you have to have the strength and resolve to be the *real* you, and if that means ending this "false" friendship, so be it.

Authentic communication should also be practiced when you meet someone now. Religious and political differences are common, and just agreeing with someone for the sake of it is inauthentic. Don't get me wrong, there are many points of disagreement to account for, but these two are often-observed examples. A decent discussion is definitely possible, of course, including one that involves the authentic you and the authentic them, to boot. Remember that being authentic does not mean either being blunt or offloading our emotions. It doesn't give you permission to hurt someone's feelings. Often, things—like the truth itself—don't have to be spoken aloud. Authenticity is about understanding how we feel *in the moment*. On that note, let's examine some tactics for maintaining authentic communication:

- Be aware of your posture and make eye contact.

  - On some occasions, being authentic may involve saying something that the other person doesn't want to hear. You still have to be assertive—in a polite way—but you also have to think of your best interests. Stand or sit with an open posture, and make sure you look the other person in the eyes.

- Speak simply and clearly.

  - Beating around the bush never works. Know what you want to say, and do it in a simple manner, making everything as clear as possible.

- Keep your goal or goals in mind.

  - Remember to go into a conversation knowing what you want to get out of it, and this goes back to being true to yourself.

Authenticity is not reserved for difficult situations—it applies to *all* situations. I don't want you to be too brash, though, and adopt the attitude that if people don't like the real you, then they're not worthy of your time. Indeed, being rude, interrupting, or dominating conversations can be avoided while still maintaining authenticity. It's also important to listen authentically, and you can do so by taking some of the approaches below:

- Focus on what the other person is saying, instead of waiting for your next chance to speak. You want to take in everything that they're saying, and while it's a human trait to get ready to reply before the end of the point of discussion, you should try to avoid doing so.

- Don't interrupt, unless you need to because you're confused, lost, or need clarity on something that the other person has said. If you need to interrupt, do so politely by saying something like, "I'm sorry to stop you, but I didn't quite understand X, Y, or Z. Could you repeat that part?" That is a perfectly polite and acceptable way to interrupt, without compromising your authenticity as a listener.

- Try to phrase your words in helpful ways, such as "I was confused when you said that," as opposed to, "You confuse me." There is a huge difference here, as using "I" and not "you" sentences avoids placing blame.

- Use a suitable tone of voice to guide your understanding, and offer sympathy or compassion when called for. If you have an idea of what they felt, or how they were affected, you can identify with them in a more authentic manner.

When it comes down to it, you should always aim to show both respect and engagement in your discussions. If you show your authentic self while speaking—as well as while listening—then you heighten the chances of an all-around good experience taking place. Showing authenticity and receiving it back leads to a certain type of fulfillment, and as people, we all need to feel fulfilled. Indeed, when you're authentic, you bring your *whole* self into every interaction.

Now, authentic communication doesn't mean saying *everything* that's on your mind. The more effective approach is to evaluate what needs to be conveyed to the other person.

Mindful Communication

This isn't all about being present and focused, but those are obviously still parts of mindful communication. When you communicate mindfully, you're able to strengthen relations and become better at interacting in social settings. Your mental health will also be boosted, and we can't forget the increase in confidence levels. In addition, mindful communication can boost one's mood in the short term, such as while engaging in communication, and in the long term, too, such as during time spent away from situations involving communication. With that said, let's turn our attention to some methods of mindful communication:

- Show gratitude and forgiveness.

  ○ You may be grateful for a friendship or just for something a friend's done for you. As such, it's always a good idea to *express* your gratitude. This makes the other person feel appreciated, and even if they didn't expect you to voice your gratitude, they'll be pleased to receive it. Furthermore, holding onto grudges is bad for you, so make no mistake—

forgiveness is always your best option. It can be difficult to forgive, and if reconciliation follows, it may take time, but if you're sincere, you'll be able to patch things up and move forward.

- Apologize when you need to.

  ○ There are times when you're 100% right, but perhaps you've still upset somebody. In cases like this, you don't need to emphasize *why* you're right. Instead, you can offer a simple apology, such as, "I didn't realize that I would hurt you when I said A, B, and C, but now that I have, I'd like to apologize." That's succinct, polite, and mindful. Well done!

- Be conscientious.

  ○ This is a form of awareness in that you want to communicate compassionately while being mindful of the other person. You also need to be conscientious of the things you say and the ways you act, so as to make sure they're not harmful to others.

- Be open and honest.

  ○ If you disagree, then say so. If you have done something wrong, tell the truth about it instead of lying and trying to hide aspects of that thing. Honesty can result in uncomfortable situations, but to respect the other party, you have to be open and honest while accepting the consequences.

  ○ Again, remember to use "I" statements, as in "I felt hurt," or "I felt neglected," as opposed to "You hurt me," or "You neglected me."

- Don't jump to conclusions.

  o This is one of the easiest things to do, and at this point, let me remind you of the cautionary tale of the snake and the belt from Chapter 4. For a quick recap, the snake (a scary thing) turned out to be a belt (a not-scary thing). So, you need to take the same logic and apply it to your conversations now. In short, listen to everything before making up your mind. While a discussion is ongoing, you never know the twists, turns, and eventual outcomes ahead of time. So, have patience, and draw your conclusions only when you have all the information.

- Create your own boundaries, and don't cross other people's.

  o If you're uncomfortable with a topic of discussion, or if you don't like greeting people with a hug, then make this known to the other person. You should expect the same back, and when everyone knows where they stand, communication can flourish in a more mindful way.

- Don't take things too personally.

  o Often, we take offense when we really shouldn't. So, think about whether it's worth being personally affected because, honestly, most times it really isn't.

Making Big Decisions

With a clearer mind, as obtained through meditation and mindfulness, you'll be more capable of making the right decisions. In order to do so, though, you'll have to think deeply and go through all the processes that may be relevant to the decision. What follows, then, are some useful tips when it comes to your preparation:

- Ask the right questions, either aloud or in written form. Here are some examples:
  - What are my options?
  - What are the pros and cons of each option?
  - How many possible outcomes could there be?
  - How will I deal with those possible outcomes?
    - Ask these questions in an order that takes you through each step, logically and completely.
- Wait and reflect.
  - Don't rush the process. When you've made the decision already, give it 24 hours and then *revisit* that decision. If you still feel it's the correct one, then go ahead and make it.
  - If you feel some doubt, or think that you may want to look at another option, then feel free to do so.
  - If it's a bid decision, you want to get it right. If you have time, make smart use of it.
- Ask for advice.
  - Friends and family are there to offer you advice. If you feel you need it, then ask them.
  - If you feel that you don't, ask anyway to see if the advice confirms your decision.
  - Take the advice or leave it, but in the latter situation,

make sure everyone knows it, so they don't take offense.

- ○ Close your eyes, put your hand on your heart, and ask, "What do I need to do next?" or, "Is there anything to know?"

Chapter Takeaway

Being authentic in a society that expects inauthenticity is quite an achievement, and it's something that many of us need to work on. As such, mixing compassion and mindfulness can help you get to know yourself better, which, in turn, will increase your ability to be authentic. Furthermore, you need to be kind to yourself—and to others—under the principle of common humanity. Criticizing oneself is too common, and doesn't allow for positivity. By reframing your self-criticism, though, you can disassociate from negativity, and use your would-be criticisms to learn and grow. You can also benefit from reflection, which is an easier task when meditation is employed. We've also discussed how when making big decisions, you should take your time, ask yourself the right questions, take advice, and trust your heart. And on the topic of decision-making, I believe you've made the right one by deciding to explore meditation. So, why don't we truly investigate the relationship between men and meditation next? See you in the next chapter!

CHAPTER 7:

The Bond Between Men's Health and Meditation

—◆—

The thing about meditation is you become more and more you.
–David Lynch

David Lynch, the famed filmmaker, musician, and visual artist, was clearly trying to reinforce my point in his quote above. Well, one of my points, anyway. But what I'm getting at is that the self-discovery that comes with meditation—and of course, mindfulness—is constantly making you more authentic, or at least giving you the tools to get there. With that in mind, this chapter is going to be largely about the benefits of meditation and mindful practices. Meditation is associated with your state of mind, of course, and the same can be said of mindfulness—so remember that as we go on.

Men's Health and Meditation

Believe it or not, we can do something about our physical health by becoming more active and living a healthy and balanced lifestyle. Meditation definitely helps here, and at the risk of repeating myself—but out of necessity—the clarity also allows for greater *motivation*. On the mental health side, it's a bit more complicated because, in cases of chronic anxiety or clinical depression, the process can be much slower. In saying that, meditation and mindfulness are more directly related to improved mental health rather than physical health. Mindfulness, due to its variety of exercises that can be used in so many areas—and times during your day—is associated with dramatic increases in mental well-being. Considering this, let's get to the various types of mindfulness and meditation techniques that you can use for the general purposes of improved quality of life.

Stress-Relief Breathing Exercises

You may remember that back in Chapter 2, we discussed a breathing exercise specific to stress relief. Well, the exercises that follow can be used to supplement or alter that technique I taught you. Some of the breathing drills may not be for you, which is fine—but pick out the ones you like, and give them a go:.

- Box breathing
  - Also referred to as four-square breathing, this exercise works on four counts that make a hypothetical box, or square.
  - This one is a bit unusual, as it starts with an exhale, and works as follows:
    - Exhale for a count of four seconds.
    - Hold your breath in for four seconds.
    - Inhale for another four seconds.
    - Hold for four seconds... then back to the start for the next exhale.
- Alternate nostril breathing
  - This is exactly what it sounds like, and the method is as follows:

- Inhale and exhale normally until you're breathing rhythmically.

- When you're ready, use your thumb to block your right nostril, and inhale deeply through your left nostril.

- As soon as your lungs are full, use your left thumb to block your left nostril, and exhale through your right.

- Repeat the process, and as you do, you'll notice a deep sense of calm coming over you.

- Pursed lip breathing
  - Interestingly, this technique has shown benefits among people who have lung disease-associated anxiety (American Lung Association, 2023). It works as follows:

    - Get yourself into a comfortable position with your neck and shoulders relaxed.

    - With your mouth closed, inhale through your nose (not too deeply).

    - Exhale for four seconds with your lips pursed.

    - Repeat.

  - Through short inhales, this exercise gives regular boosts to the oxygen in your blood and releases more carbon dioxide than usual.

- 4-7-8 breathing
  - This type of breathing acts as a tranquilizer for the

nervous system and is excellent for stress relief thanks to the natural calm it brings.

- Sit in a chair and make sure your back is straight.

- Rest your tongue against your two front teeth (it will be here for the whole exercise).

- Exhale through your mouth. You will automatically make a similar noise to what you would while sighing.

- Inhale through your nose while you count to four, before holding your breath for a count of seven.

- Exhale through your mouth for eight seconds.

- You can pause and go back to natural breathing for a few seconds, or you can go straight into round two and repeat the loop for five minutes.

- Mindful repetition breathing

  - Because mindfulness is about presence, repeating a phrase that describes your breathing can facilitate a distraction from your stress.

  - As you breathe in, you could say something like, "inhale, relax," and then, when you breathe out, you could say, "exhale, relax." Get creative if you wish, but as long as you say something that helps you stay present, you're good to go.

- Lion's breath

  - This breathing exercise is best done alone, at least for the first few times.

  - From a comfortable position, inhale deeply through

your nose and then pause for a few moments.

○ Then, aggressively let your breath out of your mouth while making a "roarrrrr" sound.

○ It may seem strange the first few times, but the idea is to take in the oxygen, and with the release of carbon dioxide comes the release of negative energy, which mimics the animalistic nature of a lion roaring.

○ When you first start with this exercise, you might feel uncomfortable, but keep it up and you'll find comfort from putting yourself in a situation in which you initially feel discomfort.

Body Scan Meditation

This is an expansion of the very brief body scan section in Chapter 3, as you'll recall. Before we can get going, though, remember that you can access guided body scan meditations on Spotify, Apple Music, YouTube, and any other music or content-sharing platform. You don't *absolutely* need the recordings, but I would advise you to check them out–they're free, after all. Now, what follows is a common body scan meditation, offered step by step:

• Get into a comfortable position, standing or sitting.

• Breathe in slowly through your nose, close your eyes, exhale through your mouth, and repeat the process until you get into a rhythm.

• Next, feel the energy around the top of your head. Take a mental note of how it feels.

• Move down to your eyes; consider what sensations you experience when you scrunch them up, and then return them to normal.

- Notice the cool air going in through your nose, as well as its warmth as you exhale.

- In your mind's eye, trace down your neck and mentally note any feelings in the area.

- Flex your shoulders and ask yourself if there is any tension there. If there is, then try your best to relax. To achieve maximum comfort, try to feel as if you're sinking into the chair or mattress.

- Make your way down your arms to your hands.

- Wiggle your fingers and identify the feelings that you get, from the inside and the outside (some imagination is required here).

- Move to your quadriceps and hamstrings, identify any tension, and sink further into comfort as you release that tension.

- Run your mind's eye down your legs, across your feet, and onto your toes, while observing the energy as you go.

- Wiggle your toes and take note of the associated feelings.

So, that's the body scan, head to toe. You can add in other parts of your body if you like. The scan could take anywhere from a few minutes to half an hour, depending on how long you spend in each area, and how detailed your observations are.

Emotional Resilience Meditation

You know all about emotional resilience by now, but there's a dedicated meditation technique that's specifically effective when it comes to developing and maintaining emotional resilience on an ongoing basis. I'd like to share it with you now:

- As usual, get yourself into a comfortable position.

- Close your eyes, and clear your mind of any thoughts.

- Focus on an imaginary point on the wall nearest to you, or the ceiling, if you're lying down.

- In your mind's eye, be as intense as you can, and hold this internal gaze for around a minute. As thoughts arrive, acknowledge them, and then dismiss them, before refocusing.

- Visualize a scenario that calls for emotional resilience, as your focus shifts from the point on the wall. Be as clear as you can, taking into account sights, sounds, feelings, and emotions.

- When you've finished, dismiss the scenario, and return to the imaginary point for another minute or so.

- Then, visualize how you would want to act in the situation you saw in your mind's eye previously.

- When you've played that scenario out, let it go, and again, return your focus to the wall.

You're engaging in a form of problem-solving, and when you head back to the wall, what you're trying to do is shift your mind and clear it of thought. As such, I would advise you to stick with one situation per meditation session, and as you begin meditating for longer, you can add in other scenarios, whether they've happened before, or may happen in the future.

Mindful Walking Meditation

We've discussed gratitude walks previously, but as a refresher, these are where you list all the things you're grateful for, along with all the people in your life you want to show gratitude for. This time, though, *mindful* walks involve you using detailed observations to clear your mind while taking in how amazing your surroundings are. Firstly, don't take your phone with you on these walks, and secondly, try to walk in nature, if possible— even if it's just in a park.

Once you're out there walking, pick out a tree and look at the intricacies in the bark. Focus on the detail in the leaves, and how they blow gently in the wind. Draw in a deep breath and break down all the different smells you experience. Then, use your ears to hear the birds chirping, the sound of the breeze, or the excerpts of conversations between people in your vicinity. Don't forget to note the texture of the path you're walking along too. If there's nobody around, you can verbalize these things you're noticing, and this may help prompt you to look closer.

As your goal is to remain present, with your senses as the methods by which you're observing the present moment, you should also keep your mind free of thoughts. We're both well aware that thoughts are bound to pop up, but I'm sure you also know by now just what to do when they arrive in your mind: acknowledge the thought, and let it go. Simple as that.

If you're also walking for exercise, you might want to walk slowly at first, and mindfully observe your surroundings, followed by speeding up your pace for physical fitness, during which time, you'll find that your exertion naturally clears your mind. Then, at the end of the exercise portion, you can slow down again and repeat the mindful observation. In general, try to go for one of these walks three or four times a week.

Gratitude Meditation

Now, I don't want to repeat myself, but as a quick reminder, gratitude can be practiced while sitting or lying down comfortably. Just list all the things you're grateful for, along with the people whom you're grateful for. You shouldn't run out of things because you can always get more detailed about small things, such as being able to have a hot meal or the fact that you have a job. Put simply, list everything you can, and you'll notice the positivity surrounding you. Gratitude can even come in the form of getting out of a toxic relationship or quitting your job because you've found yourself in a rut.

Self-Compassion Meditation

I'll try to be specific here, but all the same, remember that you can broaden the exercise to suit your situation. So, suppose you've been broken up with and are now ruminating on all the things you did wrong in the relationship. This rumination is inevitably going to lead you to self-blame and a negativity loop, in which you punish yourself for making the wrong decisions. This is, of course, completely unhelpful.

Try to sit quietly and comfortably, get a rhythmic breathing pattern going, and break everything down as much as you can. Once you've done this, you'll now be dealing with a series of small parts, instead of all the negatives associated with the entire situation. You could also use your journal for this, but whichever method you choose, be sure to get rid of all possible distractions. Indeed, you need to approach this exercise with the intention of offering yourself compassion. There will definitely be things you could have done differently, but that's simply unavoidable. In the present, they're irrelevant because, well, you can't go back in time. So, list them, accept that there's nothing you can do now, and release them, without self-judgment.

You know what happens when you suppress the associated emotions, right? So, get everything out, either in your mind or on paper. The chances are that if your relationship ended, it was meant to end, and self-blame isn't going to help you move on. You could even relate the situation to the way you'd show compassion to a loved one if *they* were the one going through a hardship. Apply that compassion to yourself, even if it's difficult. Self-forgiveness is a tool for forward motion and personal growth, so use it appropriately.

Progressive Muscle Relaxation

The idea behind this technique is to gently activate your muscles and increase your blood flow, thereby decreasing your heart rate and blood pressure. All you need to do is get comfortable, then start with your neck. Tense the muscles up, hold for five seconds, and release. You should feel looser immediately, and after you've repeated this three times, that area will be more relaxed. Next, turn to your shoulders and upper back, and tense the muscles in the same way you did with your neck muscles. After three repetitions of five seconds each, you will feel the same feeling of relaxation. Keep doing this exercise as you move down through your major muscle groups, including your stomach, quadriceps, hamstrings, and calves. As you get more fluid with this, you'll be able to incorporate breathing, aiming to match the length of your tension and release. This exercise is very effective for general relaxation, and I always recommend its use.

Mindful Visualization

Remember S.M.A.R.T. goals? As a reminder, this is a goal-setting framework that is an excellent method for tackling any number of goals. So, let's say your goal is to get a promotion at work. Relatively specific, right? Picture the conversation with your boss, and everything that you want to happen in that moment.

Now, you're getting *very* specific, which is what you want. Next, ask yourself how you can *measure* that goal. The answer is probably by aiming for a solid performance in every task, presentation, or anything else work-related that's required. Each time you succeed, your boss will take note, and you can also visualize their reaction and the compliments you'll receive. Your goal is *achievable*—you have to believe that—and by reciting a phrase like, "Getting promoted is a big possibility," or, "I know that if I work hard I will be promoted," you can make it so. Indeed, the relevance is there already, and you can add to it by mentally listing all the current and future reasons for your impending promotion. Come up with a reasonable timeframe, and break it down into small chunks, so that you can mark your success as you reach each time check. Spend 10 minutes visualizing back and forth. You might find your mind jumping ahead or skipping steps. When it does, bring it back to neutral and pick it up at the point where you were visualizing beforehand.

Chakra Activation Meditation

No, things are not about to get strange, and chakras are likely not what you think they are. The word "chakra" translates to "wheel" or "circle," and when applied to the body, it describes a sensation point that is either the source of pain or pleasure. The idea is that these points represent the energies circulating in your body. They are like car engines that need to be in tune, with all parts working simultaneously. Life, including nonhuman life, is all controlled by energies, and you probably know what it's like to feed off someone's energy and have them feed off yours. A stand-up comedian is tasked with emitting energy through enthusiasm and animated mannerisms—they do this in order for the crowd to *feel* that energy and *return* it.

Some people don't believe in chakra, and if you're one of them, I will certainly not force chakra meditation on you, but it's something I would still suggest trying. It's believed that there are 109 chakras in the body. However, seven of them are crucial to meditation and maintaining a high level of overall energy (Art of Living, n.d.). They are as follows:

- *Muladhara* chakra (or in plain English, the root chakra associated with the color red)
    - located at the base of your spine
        - associated with inertia and enthusiasm
- *Swadishthana* chakra (or in plain English, sacral chakra associated with the color orange)
    - located behind your genitals
        - associated with creation and procreation. When this chakra gets activated, one experiences either a burst of ingenuity and creativity or excessive lust.
- *Manipura* chakra (or in plain English, solar plexus chakra associated with the color yellow)
    - located in the area around the bottom of your stomach where your ribs start
        - associated with emotions like joy, generosity, greed, and jealousy
        - As you can see, not all chakras have positive associations. That being said, it's up to you to let the negativity go and focus on joy and generosity, rather than greed and jealousy.
- *Anahata* chakra (or in plain English, heart chakra associated with the color green).
    - located in the heart regions

- associated with love and hate (again, both positive and negative)

- *Vishuddhi* chakra (or in plain English, throat chakra associated with the color blue, like the sky).

  - located next to the thyroid

    - associated with the positive of gratitude and the negative of grief

    - This is the engine that connects us with others.

- *Ajna* chakra (or in plain English, third eye chakra associated with the color indigo).

  - located in the space between your eyebrows

    - associated with anger and awareness. Bear in mind that anger is normal, but it's up to us to direct it along a positive path.

- *Sahasrara* chakra (or in plain English, crown chakra associated with the color white).

  - located in your crown (the top of your head)

    - associated with bliss and pure joy

    - This chakra acts as our connection with the divine plane or our astral plane.

In the historical pursuit of harmony and happiness, meditators have pursued the activation of *all* of the chakras, both good and bad, with the aim of dismissing the bad—or at the very least, being able to *identify* it and *remedy* it. You can see this like a body scan, with attention being paid to each point. It's not for everyone, of course, and maybe it's a bit out there, but if you so wish, give it a go. The worst that could happen is you find it's not for you, and if so, you have a plethora of other types of meditation you can use.

Never Feel Ashamed

So, we've previously talked about shame as an emotion with a trigger, as well as an emotion with no apparent source. This, then, is what often makes shame a main player in both circumstantial and clinical depression. However, right now, I'm telling you not to feel ashamed of your meditation pursuits, including chakra meditation. By now, you know full well that the traditional definition of what it means to be "a man" needs to be changed, and if you practice both meditation and mindfulness— and keep this practice a secret because you're ashamed—then you're actually part of the problem. I'm sorry to be so direct, but all I'm trying to do here is paint things the way they are.

You should feel proud that meditation and mindfulness are part of your life. Indeed, you should be glad of the benefits that they offer, and pat yourself on the back for being proactive enough to allow those benefits to be enjoyed. If someone squints their eyes or turns their nose up at the news that you practice mindfulness and meditation, it's *that person* who isn't benefiting— not *you*. You should be proud enough to advertise what you have added to your lifestyle, and if you come across opposition, you should challenge those opponents to try it themselves before they make an uninformed decision.

Now, to help you along, I'm going to give you some tips on how to deal with shame. As I've said, it shouldn't be present regarding your meditation and mindfulness practice, but you can apply the tips outside of that realm too, if need be.

- Recognize shame.
    - This isn't too onerous a task because we've all felt

shame, and thus, you should know how to identify it.

- Understand the origins.

  - Perhaps you were talked down to as a child, or you were told that you were ugly or stupid, and the result has been unfounded shame. It's up to you, then, to pinpoint the origins, no matter what they may be.

- Make a point to check in with yourself.

  - This should be done in a self-compassionate way, as you explore all the reasons why you should *not* be shameful.

- Write yourself a self-compassion letter.

  - You know all about self-compassion, and you are more than capable of writing a letter to yourself. There is no need to post it, but I encourage you to read it out loud regularly, to drive the point home.

- Break it down.

  - Consider the different aspects of the shame you feel, and as with problem-solving, you can deal with those aspects better in a step-by-step process.

- Repeat your affirmations.

  - When you have all the reasons that you should not feel shame down, frame them in a set of statements that can become daily affirmations. The more you repeat them, the more truth they attract, and the less shame you will feel.

Chapter Takeaway

Whether you prefer box breathing, alternate nostril breathing, or any of the rest, I encourage you to keep the practice going. And please don't forget mindful repetition breathing! Furthermore, the body scan technique is one that you can aim to master, and I urge you to take your time, whether you're doing it on your own or while listening to a recording. Always try to remain present, and return yourself to your points of focus when your mind starts to wander. Emotional resilience, too, is a virtue that you can develop through meditation, with some visualization added to the equation. On top of that, don't forget to take a mindfulness walk and meditate in a way that enables you to feel compassion. Progressive muscle relaxation is another excellent way to align the mental and physical sides of yourself, and you can engage your chakras by following a similar method to the body scan if you wish. Lastly, let me remind you never to be ashamed of your practice, and let me also remind you to go through the steps to deal with shame outside of meditation and mindfulness. These pursuits are about empowerment, and I want you to keep that in mind as we now explore empowerment in the final chapter. Follow me!

CHAPTER 8:

Quick Tips for Empowerment

—◆—

Champions come and go, but to be legendary, you got to have heart, more heart than the next man, more than anyone in the world.
–Muhammad Ali

Ali really was the greatest, wasn't he? You may not be seeking legendary status in boxing—or any sport for that matter—but if you have the heart, you can make yourself a legend in your own life. I'm sure you'd agree with me when I say that attaining "legendary" status is something quite rare and, of course, empowering. Keeping this thought in mind, our final chapter here is going to find us wrapping up our discussion of mindfulness and meditation by going over a set of actionable tips. Trust me, guided by these tips, you'll have the best chance at succeeding in your new venture. Let's get started!

Consistency Creates Habits

If you repeat the same practices day in and day out, you develop consistency. It's up to you whether those practices are positive or negative ones, though, and I'm sure you'd prefer to pursue the former. Now, I'm not only talking about mindfulness and meditation here—I'm actually talking about everything else you've learned thus far, from self-compassion to emotional resilience to your redefined version of manliness. Finding a healthy balance in life—including through exercise and healthy eating—is a way to remain consistent in a positive manner, as is self-discovery and vulnerability in the pursuit of forgiveness, both toward yourself and others.

Also, don't forget to practice consistency when it comes to goal-setting, and follow the S.M.A.R.T. approach no matter how big or small your goals are. By repeating the framework across all other areas of life, you are consistently cultivating positivity and will feel the mental health benefits, without a doubt. Make no mistake, when habits join together and become routines, you are in the midst of consistency. And I urge you to carry it on as, well, *consistently*, as possible. Think about it this way: If you consistently save money by putting away a decent—but not exorbitant—amount each month, then by the time you reach retirement, you will have built up a decent sum of money, and that is all thanks to consistency. I trust you can see how important this is!

Give yourself an easy start by getting a recording of a five-minute body scan or meditation routine. If you reach the point where you lose concentration, then stop the session, but come back to it the next day to maintain that consistency. In this context, you can show self-compassion whenever you start thinking you're not committing well enough to meditation.

Start Small

As the saying goes about eating an elephant, one bite at a time, the same logic is applicable to meditation and mindfulness. It is not realistic to expect to be able to meditate for 30 minutes without intrusive thoughts, within a month of starting. You also can't think that you will perfect the body scan in a week. They both take practice, and the same goes for everything you learned in the preceding chapters. Remember that you will always be bad at something before you are good at it. You know this, because you have had to learn how to do things in life, and when you first start, an expectation of excellence is unfounded. If you learned to play the piano as a child, you were bad at the start and practiced to the point where you could string three chords together. You practiced more, and before you knew it, you were writing songs. Take sports, your first free throw, touchdown pass, or shot at goal, probably didn't go well, but in small steps, you improved, until you developed your all-around game. Sometimes, things seem difficult, and that is because you are looking at them as a whole. Your improvement was slow, and in small steps, but inevitably, you got to the medium-sized steps, and then the big steps. The aforesaid should be a lesson, and achieving small meditation and mindfulness goals, all operate as steps in pursuit of the ultimate goal. The hardest part is starting, the second hardest part is developing a routine, and then comes the easy part of maintaining it as all the small steps come together, and remain together.

Experience

Honestly, nothing about the actual practice of meditation is too strict to comply with. It's a means of relaxation, which allows for some experimentation. You are well within your rights to alter a breathing exercise or combine two of them to develop a technique that works best for you. On the topic of breathing, though, it's possible to find yourself out of breath in certain exercises. This isn't hugely common, but nonetheless, you need to be aware that if you're feeling out of breath, then that particular exercise is most likely not for you.

There is so much to interpret when it comes to mindfulness, and the beauty is that you have no restrictions. Deep observation can work on so many levels, from traffic to nature to sensory experiences, and you should definitely add, subtract, modify, or reinvent the exercises you've learned about. Also, try to take into account that mindfulness can be done in a wider array of places than meditation. So, don't let it be the same every time; mix it up so it doesn't get stale.

Indeed, experimentation—and your own tastes, in general—will determine how you go about your habits, which are bound to enhance your overall mindful and meditative experience. Perhaps journaling doesn't work for you. In that case, you could make an adjustment by drawing instead of writing. The artistry is not the important part here—just keep self-expression and the release of emotions at the forefront.

Another experimental idea is to combine a mindful walk with a gratitude exercise. So, every time you examine the details of your sensory experiences, think of something you're grateful for. The subject of your examination could be the very thing that you're grateful for, or it could be something completely unrelated. Whether one or the other, the combination will most likely succeed as an experiment.

Embrace Mistakes

The word "embrace" is an interesting, yet appropriate term, and it usually refers to giving someone a hug, of course. When it comes to mistakes, though, you're not quite *hugging* them. Rather, you're just not hiding them or refusing to think about them.

Now, you know as well as I do that nobody has ever gone through life without making a mistake. We all make thousands upon thousands—some small, some big. We can't let them eat us up, nor can we ruminate about how we should have acted differently. It's always easier to decide the best course of action retrospectively. The point is, people are not that unique when it comes to making mistakes, and this is why you need to identify them, accept them (*embrace* them), and release them in a way that allows you to learn, grow, and do better next time. Think back to Thomas Edison—he didn't see his 1,000 attempts as failures, but rather mistakes that he learned from in the ultimate pursuit of success.

Set Goals

It's easy to set goals, but it's even easier not to. You may think that all your goals are neatly organized in your mind, and you're very familiar with them, but until you formally *set* them, they are not really that achievable. Of course, we've already gone over S.M.A.R.T. goals quite a bit, but really, I only mention them again because of how ideal and widely applicable they are. They're a practical means to set achievable goals, then achieve them, and move to the next goal.

If your goals are going to be S.M.A.R.T., though, they need to have a time stamp. As you'll recall, I referred to irritability previously, and your hypothetical efforts to reframe it. Well, that can be turned into a goal by cutting down on your displays of irritation by, say, half. You then have a frame of measurement by simply counting your outward displays of irritation. Getting to the point where you show no irritation, and even further—to the point where you don't feel it anymore at all—then you've succeeded. Now, I realize that the "S" in "S.M.A.R.T." stands for specific, but that doesn't mean there can't be goals that are slightly more general, as opposed to the specific end of the spectrum. Ideally, you should write them down, and name them every day, so it becomes a habit.

Integration

Another term that's open to interpretation, but that I'm sure we would agree is one of the foremost in meditation and mindfulness, is *integration*. What I'm talking about here are close relationships overlapping each other. Integration can also refer to the ways in which you integrate meditation and mindfulness into your life. One would hope that the stereotypes and myths have been dismissed by now, and because of that, the integration of the two practices is neither a stereotype, nor a myth, but a genuine reflection of integration.

We can even take the idea of integration further by looking at all the different meditation and mindfulness exercises available. One can flow into the other, and the integration can become a synergy that has a positive knock-on effect over all other areas of your life. Think about it: You could practice mindfulness as part of your morning routine. Smell the coffee... no, *really* smell the coffee, taking in all its aromas. Enjoy your shower as an experience. Focus on the warm droplets hitting your back, the way they run down your shoulders, and the whirlpool motion that they make as they slide down the drain. Massage your scalp when you wash your hair, and feel the shampoo in great detail with your hands. Take heed of the way the towel feels as you dry yourself, and the sensations that your clothes leave on your skin as you get dressed. Maybe you meditate in the mornings, and if so, you can integrate the meditation into the mindful preparation for your day. Your commute should also be a mindful one, and when you reach your desk, you might even want to do a breathing exercise before you start working. By doing all these things, you are deepening the integration of mindfulness and meditation into your day-to-day life.

Self-Compassion

Yes, we've already talked about this, but it deserves another special mention. Show yourself the same kind of compassion that you would show to a loved one if they were in the same circumstances. Like all of us, you don't have long on this planet, so be as kind to yourself as possible. Don't give yourself a free pass, but more importantly, cast off the judgment, and be more delicate with yourself.

As you may remember me saying, we are our own harshest critics, and this is why you should start holding back on that criticism and using adverse experiences as learning opportunities.

See them as challenges you can learn from. A breakup or divorce can act as a trigger for self-criticism and a lack of self-compassion. You may see yourself as the problem, or the reason for the breakdown in the relationship. This is a classic example, of course, but I want to reaffirm that it wasn't all your fault, and furthermore, that the parts that *were* your fault cannot be changed. So, take a step back and show yourself the compassion that you deserve, because you *do* deserve it.

Please bear in mind that the end of a relationship is a very practical example, but it isn't only in that context that you need to show yourself some compassion. If you have made a bad decision, that's okay—so have we all. As such, remember to accept your mistakes, but still be compassionate enough to acknowledge them, learn from them, and dismiss them so that you can move forward and grow *as a man*. Self-compassion doesn't make you weak, or soft, or not willing to stand up and admit that you have acted in error. Rather, it prompts you to learn, rectify, and move forward.

Connections

Whether you are shy or confident, an introvert or an extrovert, we all need human connections. Some more than others—of that, I have no doubt—and meditation and mindfulness together can help you grow connections and improve your relationships. Never forget that you have a support system, and your connection with each person in it is different. Sure, there are bound to be some similarities, but no *one* human connection is the same as the next. In addition to human connections, there is the mind and body connection that you know all about by now, along with the various connections between mindfulness, meditation, and effective day-to-day operation.

Meditation brings with it a sense of calm and clarity, and these qualities alone can aid our connections—or reconnections—

with people we have not been in touch with in a long time. You shouldn't take any relationship for granted, and wherever you feel that gratitude should be displayed, you should absolutely display it in that area. By telling a person you appreciate that you, well, *appreciate them*, this is an act of strengthening that connection. Suppose you have been out of contact with a former friend for a decade. You can't call that person a friend because of just how long that absence has been, right? But wouldn't it be great if you could get in contact again, and truly reconnect? Of course it would, and there is nothing stopping you from reaching out and reigniting that friendship flame. And who knows, perhaps meditation and mindfulness could help revive that relationship, and you could both share in a passion for it together!

Mindful Breathing

Before we get into this section, I want you to keep in mind that when things get complicated, you can take some resting time, and even realign with some elongated breathing exercises.

I mention mindful breathing here because I would like to reaffirm its importance. Breath control and breathing exercises together have a tremendous set of benefits, which are enhanced all the more with the addition of mindful breathing. Let me remind you to experiment because, yes, to a certain degree, mindful breathing can be experimented with. It isn't especially difficult to regulate your breath, and when you do, you can synchronize your inhales and exhale with whatever mindfulness exercise you are doing at the time.

If we take positive affirmations in the form of statements, either internally or out loud, we can combine a positive assertion with an inhale, and the dismissal of a negative influence through an exhale. The body scan doesn't specifically call on rhythmic breathing, but many recordings will start by guiding you through the breathwork that you should do in preparation for the body scan. You can check in with yourself several times a day to see if you have been doing deep breathing exercises. It's quite possible that you haven't had the chance because you've been busy at work, but when you get a short amount of time to yourself, you should try to engage in one or more of the breathing exercises we've discussed.

Also, part of mindfulness is deep focus, and so if you have the opportunity, you should *live* the experience of the coolness over your nostrils as you inhale, and the warmth around your lips as you exhale. If the 3-7-8 technique works for you, then you should practice it mindfully, and be specific about your observations—both physical and mental. Everything else aside, it's not the exercise or the execution that needs to be the main focus, but rather, it's exercising mindfulness in a manner that's tailored to you that matters, even if it's a step away from meditation.

Visualization and deep breathing also fit well together and can incorporate mindfulness in two contexts. When you are engaging in mindful visualization, try to direct your attention to the sights taken in by your mind's eye, rather than the breathing. It's probably best to be aware of your breathing too, of course, but just restrict it to one of the simpler techniques. Alternatively, find a rhythm that aligns with whatever it is that you're visualizing.

Celebrate

This could also be called "success," but the end result is that you should *celebrate* success. Indeed, you should celebrate as part of your progression through mindfulness and meditation, but also any other success that comes your way. You don't have to throw a huge party or anything, but where you aimed to do well—and you did—then you deserve a pat on the back.

When it comes to the smaller things, self-congratulation without a ceremony works well, but for something big, like a promotion, the streamers and balloons should come out. With each landmark, you have achieved something, and to motivate you to put in the work to hit the next mark, you need to self-congratulate, understand that you're worthy of praise, and when you have praised yourself, you then need to turn your focus to the next sub-goal, along the path to the overall goal. Celebrating sends a signal to the brain that *yes*, you did well, and now your brain can get ready for the next one.

On the more specific side, achieving your meditation goals—such as five minutes without mental distraction—or perhaps your mindfulness goal of a flawless body scan, is certainly deserving of self-praise. You (hopefully) have some loved ones to celebrate with when you achieve your goals, and you should absolutely do so. Your goals determine the extent of your self-praise, and whether you intend to seek praise from others or not. By the way, there is nothing wrong with seeking praise from others in your inner circle. Those who deserve your praise will be more than willing to extend their praise your way, I'm sure!

Chapter Takeaway

When it comes to striving for consistency, you can't go wrong. And the more you practice mindfulness and meditation on a consistent basis, the quicker they will become routines that form good habits. You don't have to have grandiose expectations, either—in fact, I recommend you start small. Just because you're taking steps to get where you want to go, this doesn't mean you shouldn't experiment.

Mindfulness and meditation, although they address serious issues, need not be rigid and void of interpretation. As a result, mixing, matching, adding, and subtracting are highly recommended. On top of that, you should always leave the door open to different possibilities, while also not forgetting to acknowledge your mistakes, address them, and then dismiss them when you have a clearer path toward growth.

Remember: Goal-setting is within your new skill set, and the S.M.A.R.T. framework is the best approach here, no matter how big, small, extreme, or innocuous one of your goals is. As we also discussed, the beauty of mindfulness and meditation lies in their integration, including their integration specifically into your day-to-day life. Just try your best to be compassionate with yourself in the same way you would with a friend or family member.

Human connection is something that we all need, and to that end, I encourage you to use meditation and mindfulness to give yourself the clarity you need to maintain existing connections, develop new ones, and possibly even revive former ones. To change track, I would be remiss if I didn't mention mindful breathing once more. I know I've done so several times already, but that's just because I truly want you to explore the benefits.

Finally, as this last chapter draws to a close, I would like to remind you of your power of celebration, be it small, medium, or large. And on that note, it's time to draw this chapter, and this book at large, to a close. But before I do, let's wrap things up in the Conclusion, reflecting on some of the key lessons we've learned. See you there!

CONCLUSION

—◆—

Here we are—you've made it to the end. Well done, my friend! What were your favorite parts? Have you tried any meditation or mindfulness practices yet? If so, how did they go? If you could answer these questions for me, as well as leave any comments as part of a review, I would sincerely appreciate it. I hope you have enjoyed reading this book as much as I enjoyed writing it. And if you would like to refresh your knowledge—and supplement it—do have a look at the references following this conclusion.

Now, as you proceed into a life of meditation and mindfulness, I urge you not to delay. Before you know it, a week has gone by and you haven't started. And at that rate, the unfortunate thing is you probably never will. There is no time like the present, so why not begin with some breathing exercises today? You have a lot to choose from, so feel free to give one a go, and if you decide it's not for you, then just move on to the next one.

You could also start with mindfulness, of course, right where you are sitting. For instance, you could either picture objects in your mind or pick out the details of those around you. Another option is to take out your journal and write about the people and things you're grateful for. Why not cook a meal, and focus on the smells while you do, then eat without distractions, picking apart the different flavors? Try to harness pure enjoyment, while being present in the moment—you know the drill. Get up and go for a slow walk, look at your surroundings, and focus on the detail in what you see. The body scan is a good exercise too, so maybe get YouTube up, find a recording (I would advise five minutes to start), and give it a go. Again, all I ask is that you do not delay!

I hope—and I am confident in that hope—that your opinion of

"being a man" has now been broadened. I would encourage you to think long and hard about what "being a man" means to you. Something else I hope is that you agree that toxic masculinity needs to be questioned. I'm sure that if you consider yourself a toxic male, you will change. In fact, I implore you to do so.

Forgiveness, and the ability to forgive others—and yourself—is another subject that warrants repeating. I want you to remember that holding onto resentment, or any of the other emotions that come with a reluctance to forgive, is a means to harming your own mental health. And the power of meditation can transform you by lightening your load when you apologize when you're wrong, and forgiving when you're right. Just don't place too much emphasis on being right, of course.

You are now also aware of the myths surrounding masculinity, and whether you considered meditation a women's pursuit before, I am certain that your mind has been changed. If you thought that meditation and success were unrelated, I know unequivocally that your mind has been changed. If they can use meditation for success, then so can you.

Use your masculine energy to take on the meditation and mindfulness challenge. Your problem-solving skills, your creativity, and your independence will all be improved. As you know, these are all traits of masculinity, and as they are improved upon, so, too, will your logic, and your internal strength. As a man, you need to be resilient. And sometimes, to be resilient, you first have to be vulnerable, and this goes back to stepping out of your comfort zone. Indeed, you must become *uncomfortable*, and as a result of the experience, you will become *comfortable*.

In terms of goal setting, please don't overlook the S.M.A.R.T. framework, as the method will make you even more goal-oriented, especially due to your ability to measure progress. The more you achieve, the more you will want to achieve, and S.M.A.R.T. goals will help you get there. Goals turn challenges into opportunities, which is why you have goals for your meditation and mindfulness practices too. Being able to reach five minutes of uninterrupted meditation is tough, but you will get there if you set it and monitor it as progress toward that five-minute mark. Regarding mindfulness, your goal might be to do the whole body scan without thoughts creeping in; that too is difficult, but again, you will get there.

You deserve self-compassion, so please practice it. Remember not to be too hard on yourself, and adopt the "be compassionate to myself in the same way that I would be compassionate to a friend" approach. And what comes with it? Yes, self-reflection, which is best done in your journal. Self-reflection can be a tool for improved communication in a mindful way.

You now know how to combat stress, but don't forget to pay attention to the stress relief exercises in Chapter 7. Be consistent, start small, and don't be afraid to experiment and improvise. After all, meditation is adaptable, and so is mindfulness. Finally, have fun, and celebrate every success that you find through your new pursuits of the mind—and body.

Gosh, our time has come to an end, but I would like to leave you with one final quote. You've heard it before, but I feel that's applicable to the point where you need to hear it again. Please take it to heart, and good luck on your meditation and mindfulness journey.

No matter what you do, mindfulness is something that can get you ready for the moment, no matter how big or how small it is. Even if you're not trying to hit a game-winning shot in the NBA Finals, it's important to stay centered throughout any journey so that you can enjoy it all, and not just at the end of a big moment. Often, when people focus on the outcome instead of the process, they find themselves at the end asking, "Wow, is that it? And what now?" That's a difficult situation to be in. But if you're mindfully aware of all the moments up until that point, you won't get so stuck on what was or what could be. —Michael Jordan

All areas of life...

SUMMARY

This section is dedicated to summarizing the different meditation exercises available for personal growth, health, and emotional resilience. With this handy chart, you have them all in one place and can refer back to them whenever you'd like.

General Well Being

Type of Medication	Summary
Breathing Meditation	Get into a comfortable position. Close your eyes. Breathe in deeply for a count of four. Pause for a moment. Exhale for a count of four. Aim for five minutes. Remember to focus on your breathing. When thoughts enter your mind, dismiss them, realign, and carry on.

Type of Medication	Summary
Affirmation meditation	From a comfortable position, regulate your breathing without counting. As you do so, recite affirmations regarding what you would like to implement in your life.

Emotional Resilience

Type of Medication	Summary
Exposure meditation	Sit or lie down comfortably. Close your eyes and regulate your breathing. Visualize a situation in which you were emotionally triggered. By doing so, you are slowly exposing yourself to that situation. This meditation will help you understand that it wasn't that bad. It will also teach you how to act differently in the future.

Type of Medication	Summary
5-4-3-2-1	With your eyes closed, picture five things you can see. Then, notice four things you can feel, three things you can hear, two things you can smell, and one thing you can taste. This is also called "grounding meditation," and it aims to center you and bring a sense of calm.

Type of Medication	Summary
Object focus	Again, get into a comfortable position. Close your eyes and focus on an object of your choice in your mind. Whatever you choose, make sure to be very specific about it as you make your observations. When your thoughts wander, simply acknowledge this, and realign.

Type of Medication	Summary
Alphabet/name exercise	For this exercise, you can either keep your eyes open or closed. Engage your concentration by either reciting the alphabet backward or thinking of both a male and female name that starts with each letter of the alphabet.

Type of Medication	Summary
Body scan	Get comfortable and close your eyes. From head to toe, focus on each part of your body. Note the feelings and sensations as you make your way down and then back up.

Physical Well Being

Type of Medication	Summary
Mindful walking	Simply take a slow walk, and acutely observe everything you see, feel, hear, touch, and taste. Take special care to be as specific as you can when analyzing these things through your senses.

Type of Medication	Summary
Gratitude meditation	This isn't strictly a form of meditation, and it can be done in any environment. In your mind, or on a piece of paper, list all the

	people and things that you are grateful for in your life.
Type of Medication	**Summary**
Self-compassion meditation	Get comfortable. Close your eyes. Visualize and analyze all the good things about yourself. Then, think about what you can improve on, and come up with ideas to do so.
Type of Medication	**Summary**
Progressive muscle relaxation	This isn't meditation, per se, but it works. Get as relaxed as possible, then tense up your muscles, before releasing them again. As you do, try to focus on your breathing for ultimate relaxation.
Type of Medication	**Summary**
Mindful visualization	You can use this one to focus on your S.M.A.R.T. goals. From a comfortable position, with your eyes closed, slowly address every goal from S to T.

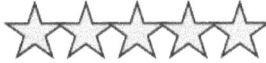

Thanks for purchasing this book.

Please support independent publishers, like me, by giving your review on amazon

https://mybook.to/meditation4men

Check out the full Meditation series

All titles in this Series include:

Introduction to Meditation

Meditation 4 Teenagers: Empowering Teens

Meditation 4 Men: Elevating Masculinity

Meditation 4 WomenOver50: Breaking Free from Menopause

Meditation 4 Grandparents (coming soon)

Meditation Coloring Book

Mindful Journal

REFERENCES

Alison Armstrong: Free listen. (n.d.). Alisonarmstrong.com. https://www.alisonarmstrong.com/free/listen.html

American Lung Association. (2023). *Pursed lip breathing.* American Lung Association. https://www.lung.org/lung-health-diseases/lung-disease-lookup/copd/resource-library/pursed-lip-breathing-video

Ankrom, S. (2023). *9 breathing exercises to relieve anxiety.* Very Well Mind. https://www.verywellmind.com/abdominal-breathing-2584115#citation-11

The Art of Living. (n.d.). *7 chakras in human body, significance & how to balance them.* The Art of Living. https://www.artofliving.org/in-en/meditation/benefits/7-chakras-significance-and-how-to-balance-them

Bates-Duford, T. (2018). *Female vs male friendships: 10 key differences.* https://psychcentral.com/blog/relationship-corner/2018/01/female-vs-male-friendships-10-key-differences#1

Blain, T. (2023). *The importance of mindful communication for your mental health.* Very Well Mind. https://www.verywellmind.com/mindful-communication-definition-principles-benefits-how-to-do-it-7489103

Brainy Quote. (n.d.). *Thomas Paine quotes.* Brainyquote.com. https://www.brainyquote.com/quotes/thomas_paine_163018

Cambridge Dictionary. (n.d.). *Synergy.* Cambridge Dictionary. https://dictionary.cambridge.org/dictionary/english/synergy

Chartier, S. (n.d.). *How men can benefit from mindfulness.* A Vogel.

https://www.avogel.ca/blog/how-can-men-benefit-from-mindfulness/

Cherry, K. (2023). *How resilience helps you cope with life's challenges.* Very Well Health. https://www.verywellmind.com/what-is-resilience-2795059

Cherry, K. (2023). *What is self-awareness?* Very Well Health. https://www.verywellmind.com/what-is-self-awareness-2795023

Cullen, K. (2022). *Suppressing emotions can harm you—here's what to do instead.* Psychology Today. https://www.psychologytoday.com/intl/blog/the-truth-about-exercise-addiction/202212/suppressing-emotions-can-harm-you-heres-what-to-do

Edwards, A. (2015). *It's a man's world: The effect of traditional masculinity on gender equality.* E-International Relations. https://www.e-ir.info/2015/03/29/its-a-mans-world-the-effect-of-traditional-masculinity-on-gender-equality/

Ferguson, S. (2022). *All about human personality: Definition, disorders, and theories.* Psych Central. https://psychcentral.com/health/what-is-personality

Gates, B. (2018). *Why I'm into meditation.* Gates Notes Blog. https://www.gatesnotes.com/The-Headspace-Guide-to-Meditation-and-Mindfulness

Gupta, S. (2023). *The importance of self-reflection: How looking inward can improve your mental health.* Very Well Mind. https://www.verywellmind.com/self-reflection-importance-benefits-and-strategies-7500858#:~:text=Ask%20yourself%20open%2Dended%20questions,anyone%20for%20granted%3F%E2%80%9D%20Notice%20what

Irene Sophia Plank et al. (2021). *Motherhood and empathy: Increased activation in empathy areas in response to other's in pain.*

ResearchGate.
https://www.researchgate.net/publication/352247397_Mot
herhood_and_empathy_increased_activation_in_empathy_ar
eas_in_response_to_other's_in_pain

Kesebir, S. (2019). *Research: How men and women view competition differently.* Harvard Business Review.
https://hbr.org/2019/11/research-how-men-and-women-
view-competition-
differently#:~:text=Past%20research%20has%20pointed%2
0to,competition%20are%20higher%20for%20them.

Jane Graney et al. (2024). *Antecedents and service contact in an observational study of 242 suicide deaths in middle-aged men in England, Scotland and Wales, 2017.* BMJ Public Health.
https://bmjpublichealth.bmj.com/content/2/1/e000319

Kubala, K. (2023). *7 tips to help in your decision making process.* Psych Central. https://psychcentral.com/health/tips-to-help-you-
make-the-most-important-decisions

Learn to communicate authentically. (n.d.). Alberta Alis.
https://alis.alberta.ca/succeed-at-work/make-your-work-
life-more-satisfying/learn-to-communicate-
authentically/#:~:text=When%20you%20communicate%20
authentically%2C%20you%20bring%20your%20whole%20s
elf%E2%80%94your,makes%20you%20feel%20more%20co
nfident.

Lovering, C. (2021). *How to practice loving kindness meditation.* Psych Central. https://psychcentral.com/health/loving-kindness-
meditation

Maharishi International University Research. (n.d.). Research.miu.
https://research.miu.edu/maharishi-
effect/#:~:text=Generally%2C%20the%20Maharishi%20Ef
fect%20may,including%20Yogic%20Flying%2C%20in%201
976.

Marsden, P. (2018). *What does it mean to be a man today?* Brand Genetics. https://brandgenetics.com/es/human-thinking/what-does-it-mean-to-be-a-man-today-2/

Mead, E. (2019). *What is mindful self-compassion? (Incl. exercises + PDF).* Positive Psychology. https://positivepsychology.com/mindful-self-compassion/

Natale, N., & Welch, H. (2023). *11 highly successful CEOs and celebrities who practice meditation.* https://www.everydayhealth.com/meditation/highly-successful-ceos-celebrities-who-practice-meditation/

Pursed lip breathing. (2023). American Lung Association. https://www.lung.org/lung-health-diseases/lung-disease-lookup/copd/resource-library/pursed-lip-breathing-video

quoteresearch. (2017). *Resentment is like taking poison and waiting for the other person to die.* Quote Investigator. https://quoteinvestigator.com/2017/08/19/resentment/

Sinusoid, D. (2021). *What causes shame? How men and women differ.* Shortform.com. https://www.shortform.com/blog/what-causes-shame-how-men-and-women-differ/

Smith, C. (n.d.). *Michael Jordan and mindfulness.* Round Glass Living. https://roundglassliving.com/meditation/articles/michael-jordan-mindfulness

Synergy. (n.d.). The Cambridge Dictionary. https://dictionary.cambridge.org/dictionary/english/synergy

Tartakovsky, M. (2011). *Cultivating self-compassion.* Psych Central. https://psychcentral.com/blog/cultivating-self-compassion#1

36 famous celebrities and successful people who meditate (The ultimate list). (n.d.). Dreamelifelab.org. https://dreamlifelab.org/celebrities-who-meditate

Waugh, R. (2018). *There really are mental differences between the sexes (and men are more analytical).* Yahoo News. https://uk.news.yahoo.com/really-mental-differences-sexes-men-analytical-142321417.html?

World Health Organization. (2023). *Depressive disorder (depression).* World Health Organization. https://www.who.int/news-room/fact-sheets/detail/depression

·